Our Brave Hearts

For Fionn and Molly, my loves.
What a gift it is to be your mother.
I will always be grateful that you chose me in this lifetime.

To Stuart,
none of this adventure would have been possible without you.
I love you more with every passing week, month, and year.

In memory of my mother, Anne Agnew,
one of the greatest loves of my life.

Our Brave Hearts

Wise Words for Mothers

Jacqueline Kelly
Illustrations by Rosie Lovelock

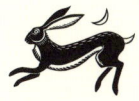

Leaping Hare Press

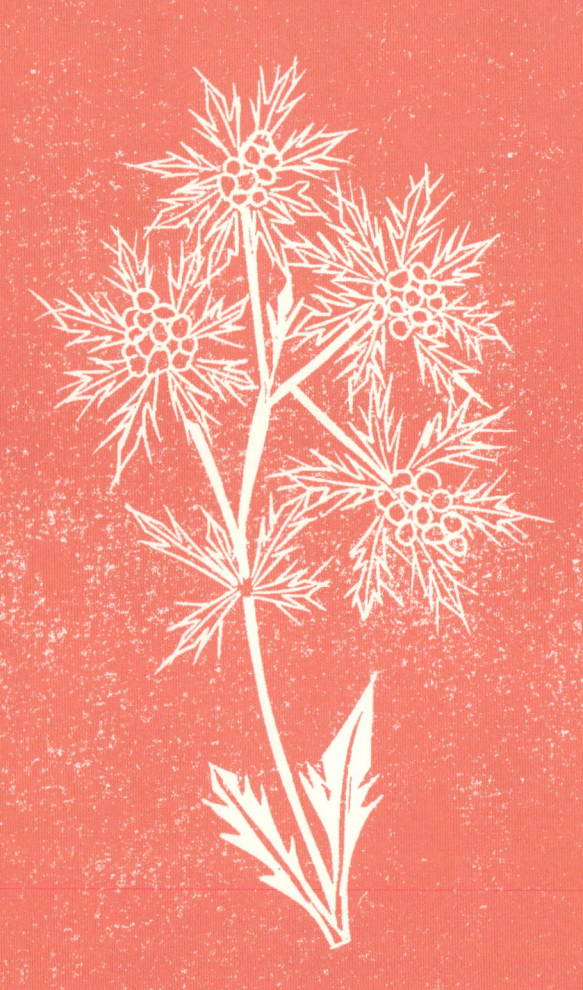

Contents

Introduction..7

The birth of a mother........................11

The act of mothering........................ 23

The grief of a mother........................51

A mother and her loved ones..........73

When I lost my self............................85

My self, my strength 113

Mental health resources....................................140

Further reading..142

About the author..143

About the illustrator..143

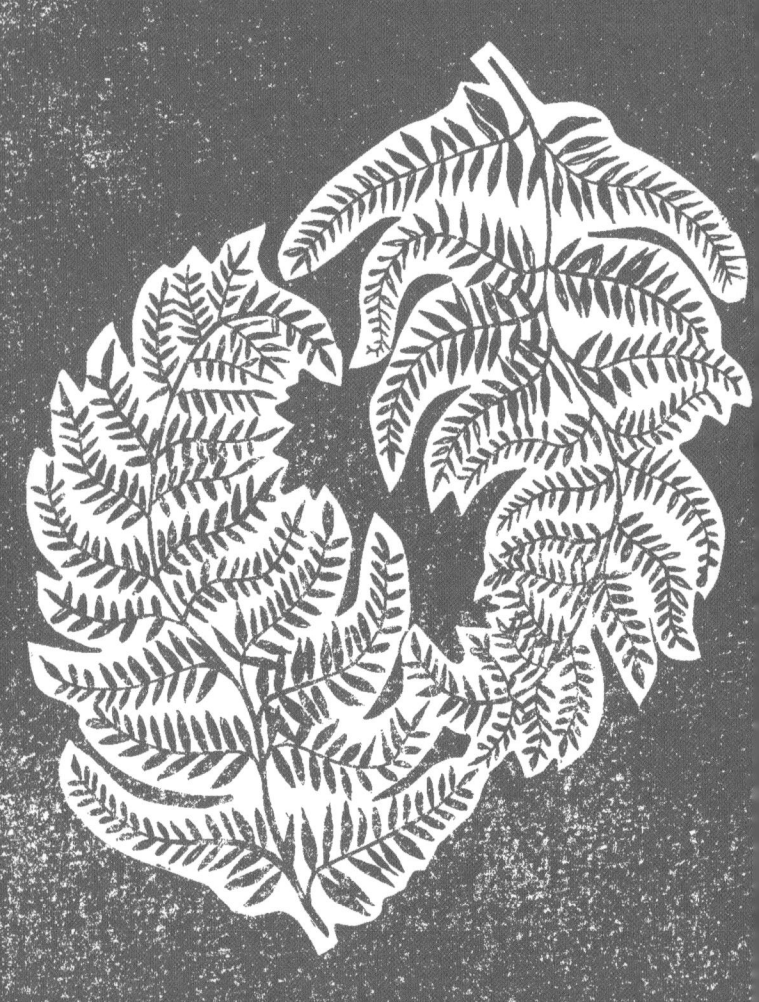

Introduction

Some people think I complain about motherhood. They tell me I moan about it as if the fact that I talk about how challenging it is somehow means I don't like it. What these people don't understand is that my motherhood was never the problem. The 'problem' was my attachment to a meaning of motherhood that wasn't true.

I have spent a great deal of my life searching. Searching for a purpose, searching for a reason why I was the way I was, searching for some sort of peace, some sort of certainty and searching for a truth that felt like my own. I imagined that there was a truth out there for me that when I found it and lived it, I would feel slide over me and settle in my bones with certainty.

I never imagined that my truth would be painful or that it would shift constantly under my feet as I changed day to day. When my first child arrived in 2013, I was not expecting to shatter into a million pieces. I didn't know that my son Fionn would become my biggest teacher.

What I have realized is that my son brought with him my purpose – a version of my truth that hurt to bear witness to and all the other things that I had spent my life searching for.

Motherhood has been for me what some people call a spiritual awakening. It has dragged me to depths of myself that I could never have imagined existed. I have had to face and question all that I knew to be true and I know now that I will never truly stand in my truth for longer than a few moments at a time because my truth, like me, is annihilated time and time again.

When I look back over my years, I can see that the times in my life where I was changing, where I was no longer one thing and not yet quite another, or where I was outgrowing one version of truth for another, these are the times in my life that the call for me to explore what I thought was possible was strongest.

As I have grown into each version of myself, painfully at first and then with complete ease and surrender at the beautiful inevitability of knowing this was where I was supposed to be, I look back and wonder at the fear that is ever present at the beginning of change. Why am I afraid of who I am becoming?

And so here I am all these years later, slowly coming round to the idea that our truths are not things to be measured – they are to be felt. I have gone from being a lover to a wife, a maiden to a mother and a soulmate of my mother to no longer having her earthside with me. Each of these moments in time, each exploration of the liminal space, has brought untold grief and joy. I have died many times in my life for me to become the woman I am today. As I birthed my son, I was unknowingly bidding farewell to the woman I had been. As I was handed my child, I breathed my last breath as the woman I was and a second later I took my first breath as a mother.

Almost two years later as I laboured with my daughter, I began the descent into grief as the mother-of-one that I had been began her withdrawal from my life. As Molly was born into water and then passed up to me, I welcomed her as my newly emerged 'mother of two' self.

When I received the news that my mother's life hung in the balance as a result of complications after surgery, I withdrew into the most painful and transformative cocoon of my life. Thirty-three days later my mother died and with her a part of me too.

I emerged from that cocoon bruised and fragile, a new version of myself that I am still getting to know.

As my soul absorbs the experiences of my life, I know that the mother role is central to who I have been, who I am and who I am becoming. Becoming a mother has changed me in ways that I still find difficult to put into words, probably because when we name it we are somehow caging it and I don't think this is a feeling that can be caged. It is too primitive, too raw and too powerful.

Just when I think I feel the words making their way from my soul to my tongue, the sands of my truth shift beneath me and I am left with words that cannot do justice to what it is I am feeling. But I still speak the words that a moment ago felt true. I release them so that I can explore what I imagine they mean. I trust that in doing so it makes space for my soul to continue showing me who it is I am becoming when I allow myself to let go of who I have been.

I receive so many different responses to my writing but one thread that runs through a lot of them would be that my writing helps mothers feel less alone. In my words, they often see the parts of their own motherhoods that they haven't been able to put into words. This book is a call for all mothers to 'complain' – to be honest with themselves and others, and experience just how liberating it can be.

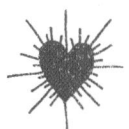
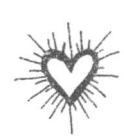

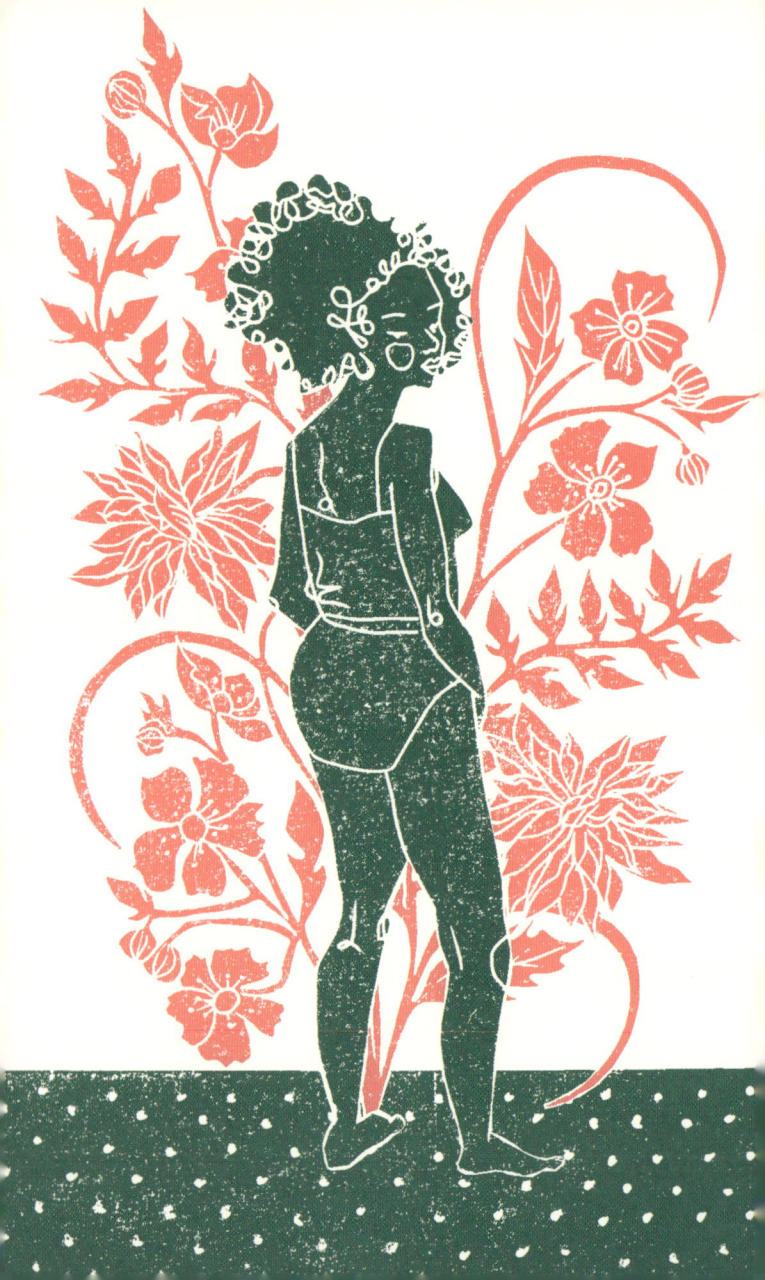

The birth of a mother

How do we navigate a world turned upside down? As I stumbled, bleeding and broken, through my first few weeks of motherhood, feelings of love made themselves known to me as I took in the perfection of the boy who was now mine for a while. Awe battled with shock and trauma. So many tears.

I spent so much time in the early weeks and months of my motherhood desperately trying to gather up the dead skin of the woman I was shedding. Who was I if not the woman I had always been? For many mothers, our experiences of motherhood have not been 'adequately contained' by the people and the societies around us.

What do I mean by this? Well, we have not been allowed to grieve and weep for the letting go of the women we were. We have been asked to contort ourselves into what other people think we should look and act like as women and as mothers. Motherhood tore my romantic ideals away from me. It left me bleeding and kneeling among the ruins of the life I had always known. I had nowhere to look but at a version of myself I no longer recognized. I had never experienced such rawness, such painful vulnerability as I did after the reckoning that is giving birth. It took time to rise from my knees.

I blamed myself for feeling like I was not succeeding at something that I believed should have come easier to me. I blamed myself for not succeeding at something society would have had me believe would come easily and naturally. I blamed myself for the feelings of emptiness that sometimes threatened to consume me. I felt like an echo chamber full of memories and images of who I had always been; I was so frightened at the idea of letting her go.

I panicked. I thought I was losing myself.

I thought I was disappearing behind the magnificence of the new life I was now responsible for. Time has taught me that I was never lost. I was just somewhere I had never been before. And it takes a beautiful surrender of the heart and mind to truly understand the difference.

The woman I was is gone. I am no longer her. But she will always be part of who I am becoming.

How was your birth, dearest mother?

To birth the mother inside of you, the one who pays no heed to what society expects and demands of her, the one who claims her place in this world in a burst of rage and hope and fierceness, and laughs in the face of a world that dares tell her she's not good enough, you must tear yourself apart.

The mother in you is both ferocious and fragile. She is as capable of destruction as she is of creation. She will walk to the ends of the earth on bloodied feet to provide safety for her children and she will stand strong and fearless in the face of anything that threatens her cubs.

Why, then, does she punish herself for not being 'good enough'? Why does she weep from wounds that are inflicted by a society that tries to fit her into a box that is too small and too narrow for such an untameable and primitive force of nature? Why, then, does she believe, even for a second, that she is failing at motherhood?

She can lift cars and bring governments to their knees to protect her child. She takes bullets for her babies and will illegally cross borders to seek protection for her little ones. She goes hungry so that they may feel full.

To become her, you have to give her permission to feel her pain. She doesn't need to be fixed. She is to be trusted and honoured as she burns to the ground every belief that has kept her chained to a paradigm of motherhood that simply does not exist. When the fires you have started are burning bright for all to see, I will come join you and dance around the flames as you rise from the ashes of the woman that society told you to be.

The mother in you is both
ferocious and **fragile**.
She is as capable of **destruction**
as she is of **creation**.

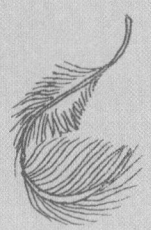
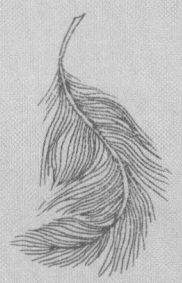

You are the only one
who gets to **define** you.
I am the only one who
gets to **define** me.
But together, we can **transform**
expectations of motherhood.
Are you **ready**?

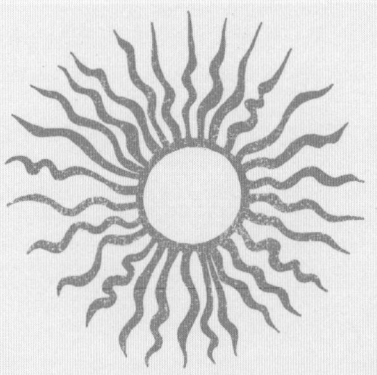

What's it like getting to know yourself as a mother?

Finding ourselves as mothers requires us to go on an epic and life-long journey. Each of us must go in search of our self, and in doing so will come up against the opinions and judgements of others. We are tested as we soul-search, and are challenged as we expand. This is the way of it. Expect no less.

When we step outside of an established way of being, we must do so with courage in our hearts – courage to keep going even when we are frightened, courage to hold space for the women who rise from the ashes with us in their own unique and magnificent ways, and courage to forge a path through the unknown wilderness even when the obstacles in our way are huge and monstrous.

We must work at letting go of our (socially encouraged) judgments of other women and our deep-rooted need for approval. This is hard work; expect no less. We must make ourselves look inwards with awe at the beauty and perfection of all that we are in this moment, and work at making this a habit until we are able to love ourselves without being reminded to do so.

It is time to cast aside the suffocating and devaluing paradigm of motherhood that society wants us to aspire to and start defining motherhood for ourselves. What makes you such a great mother? Something completely different to what makes me a great mother so why then should we compare ourselves to each other?
We may be encouraged to do so, perhaps because it is convenient in today's society to feed the toxic myth of rivalry between women. Who benefits from this? What's certain is it's not you or me.

You are the only one who gets to define you. I am the only one who gets to define me. But together, we can transform expectations of motherhood. Are you ready?

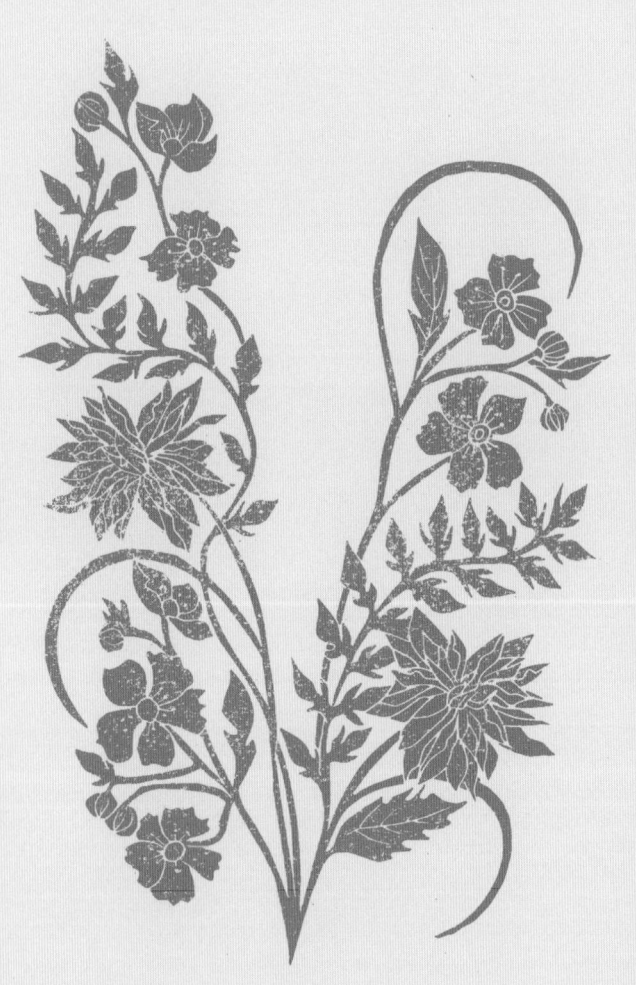

Have you ever worried that you are broken somehow?

We as mothers must learn to trust that we can be our own source of validation. We must learn to stop looking for it from others; they can only see what their life experiences have shaped them to be able to see. Their opinions of your life, your decisions and your actions need bear no weight on the trajectory of your motherhood. To appreciate that, we first have to disengage from the need to have the approval of others.

We must descend to our murky depths in order to relearn and reignite the practice of 'being' rather than living constantly in the numbing distraction of 'doing'. This may not always be a willingly undertaken journey but it is an essential and life-saving one if you are to reclaim all of who you are.

And who are you? You are someone who does not need to be fixed. You are someone to be seen and honoured as you delve into the complexities of your soul. You are someone who stops blaming, and eases with the grace of a falling feather into acceptance of all that has been and all that is. You are someone who is waking up to her true self.

This is life. This is what it means to be alive. Eventually, there will come a day when the reckoning of the soul cannot be dismissed. That day waits for you.

Did you know that you're amazing?

To add another child to your family can be scary, and you may well wonder if you'll be able to love the new baby as much as you do your first. It seemed unimaginable that I could have as deep and as wide a love for a whole new being as I did for my boy. How can a person be capable of so much love and not be destroyed in the process?

As I birthed my second child, I once again bore witness to the dying of a version of me so that the mother of two could be born. It is in these moments, the moments between my baby being nestled within me and almost being earthside, that this new emerging version of me made her way to the surface. She rose up and claimed her space, and she burnt down everything in her way so she could be born along with my daughter.

I remember these moments so vividly, as the space between contractions. It contracted and expanded so painfully, so powerfully, that I could do nothing but surrender to its force and magnitude. I remember free-falling so deeply into a knowing as old as time, a wisdom so profound that it immediately put me at ease during some of the most physically intense minutes of my life.

I knew that I was coming to the end of my labour, I knew that if I could rest for a moment, it would allow me to gather the last reserves of my strength so that I could birth my baby. I remember thinking, 'Hold on, you can do this'. My eyes were closed so that I could focus on where I had to go. It was not vision that led me but courage and conviction that soon I would be holding the baby I had spent nine months waiting to meet.

Hold on. Dig deep. Trust. Trust. Trust.

When I think of these moments, it brings tears to my eyes that I was once that woman. The woman who bravely lingered in the space between, the woman who knew instinctively when to push and when to gather her strength. I marvel at the wonder of what I experienced. As my daughter was born, so too was I as a mother of two.

The spaces between never cease to amaze me.

Hold on.
Dig deep.
Trust.

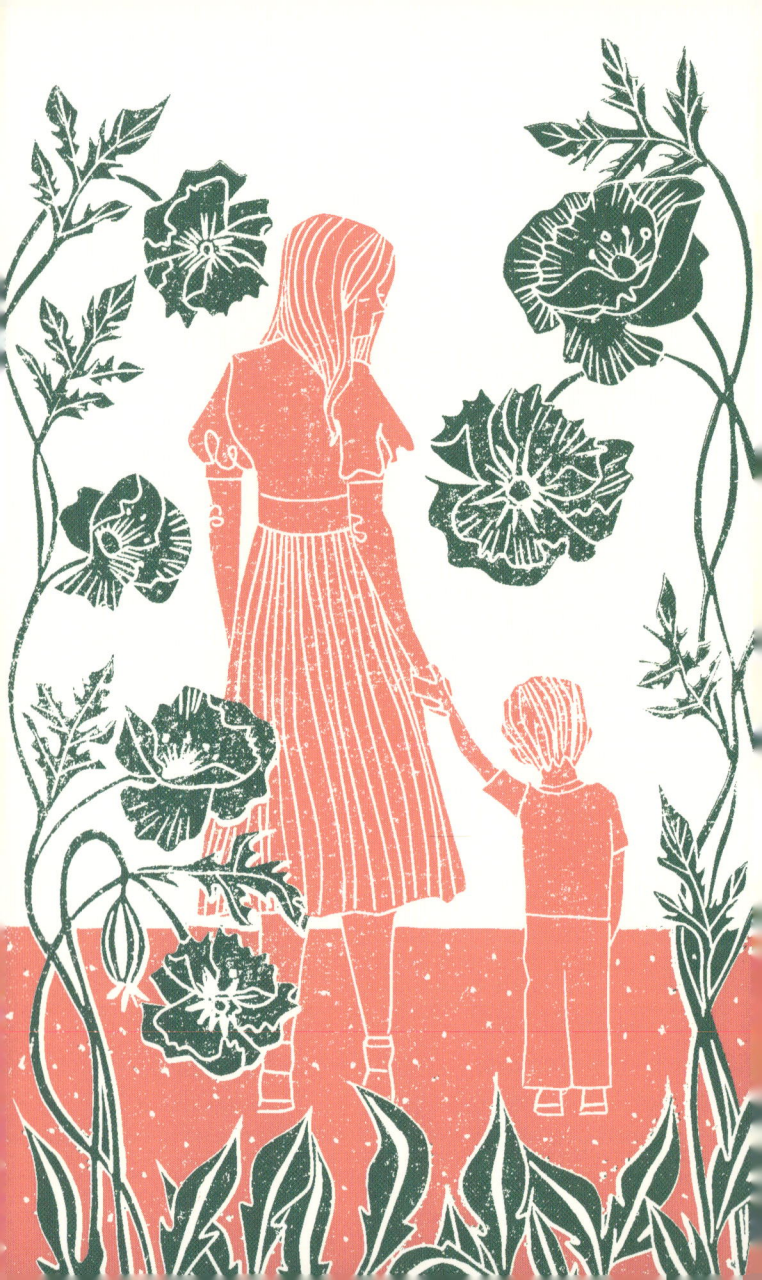

The act of mothering

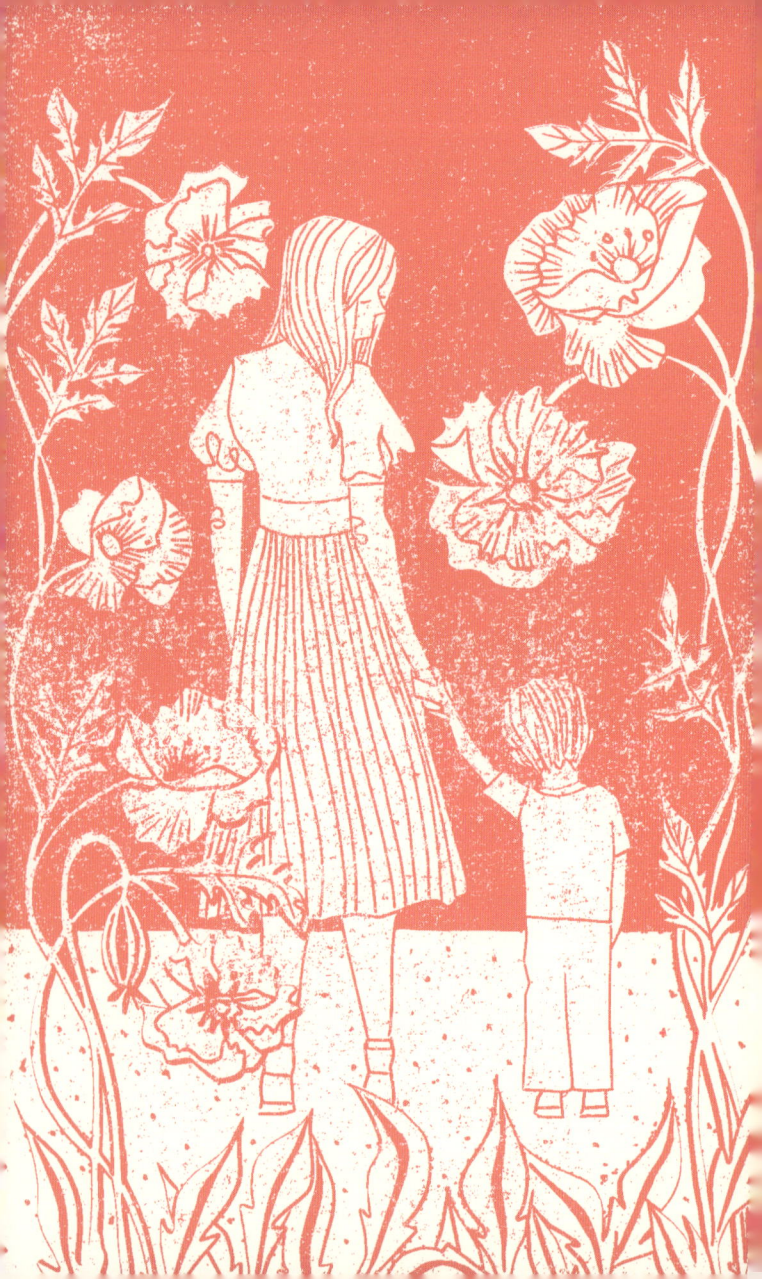

Before I became a mother, I had no idea of what it would mean to me to be a mother.

Now I know.

I am a caretaker.

A keeper of stones and all things they deem precious.

I am their lighthouse in the dark and their shelter in the storm.

I am their mother.

I am a guardian of innocence and the teacher of painful realities that are part of life.

It is me they look for when their world feels scary for it is my voice and scent they have known since before they were born.

They instinctively seek me out when they know I am around. I adore the moments when they wrap their little legs and arms around me, and when they allow the full weight of their bodies to rest upon my body. My body welcomes them home.

I am their home. I am their mother.

Their heartbeats carry the echo of mine. Forever.

When was the last time you let yourself weep with hurt?

Oh, how I could weep with frustration and hurt. A challenging day at home with the kids can be soul-destroying, especially when there have been a lot of them already. It's not like you have HR to complain to. You need to face the drudgery, day in and day out. You need to ride the wave of chaos and it can be so, so painful.

Mothering a little person through big changes in their life takes a huge amount of energy, kindness, compassion and unconditional love. There are times I question if I have it in me to do this.

It always starts off so well, I am so cool, calm and collected. My loving and calm voice is used, murmuring gentle words of reassurance and firmness. But this can only go on for so long before I want to claw my nails down a wall while roaring in rage at the futility of the situation. I bite my tongue, blood boiling.

The depth of my love for my children is infinite – my patience, not so much.

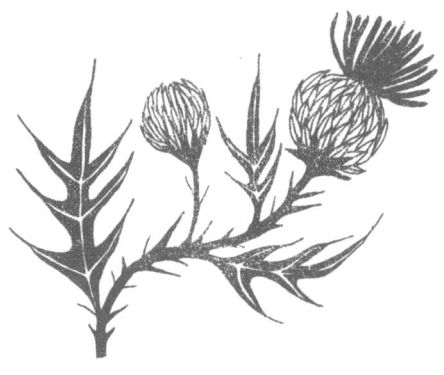

Survive.

Keep putting one foot in front of another. This too shall pass, just like all the other times passed but you've kind of forgotten just how intense and painful they were because you lived to tell the tale. I feel broken and run down in the evenings. I'm beginning to dread the late afternoon slide into evening because I know that bedtime is coming and with it, volcanic eruptions of pure emotion that rip through our home like an explosion, leaving us all spent in its wake.

I feel sad for my little one because if I am unsure of how to handle these blow-outs, I can only imagine how unsettling and scary they are for her. Her feelings are gigantic and they run her. She is in the midst of a hugely challenging time and my heart aches because I know I cannot make all of this just go away. My job is to be the container for her to implode in so that she can learn the art of shedding old layers and ways of thinking as she continues to grow and expand into the girl she is becoming.

She and I are in the trenches together right now and it is hard, it is painful and it is exhausting for us both. But when tomorrow comes, there is nowhere else I'd rather be than by her side, ready to catch her when she falls.

Sending love to all the other mothers in the trenches right now. Day by day, minute by minute, that's how we get through this.

Can you bend without breaking?

Our days are filled with ebbing and flowing, giving and taking, resisting and surrendering. We are caught in what feels like an eternal routine of learning how to bend without breaking.

How's that going for you?

I've realized that I can bend further than I ever imagined. Sometimes (most of the time) there's a lot of resistance. I often get stuck in the painful moment where I believe that somehow my children should just accept what I am telling them to do.

I believe that I'm right and I no longer see the woods for the trees. These moments are often defined by me telling rather than asking. Demanding rather than suggesting. Overbearing rather than yielding. Hard rather than soft.

I'm not bringing my children up to choke on their own opinions. It was never our intention that they would feel railroaded into doing something 'just because'. This all sounds good in theory but when you are in the thick of it and you lose sight (so quickly) of the way you intended to be, you slide straight into 'I'm the adult, you're the child. I'm right, you're wrong.'

When the heat of the moment has passed and your ego has settled down, so starts the inevitable descent into disappointment and hurt and feelings of having let yourself down. If this sounds familiar, please know you are not alone.

This is one of the murky areas of motherhood that is not

spoken about a lot because it's not all shiny with bells and whistles attached to it. It's not able to be captured in a photo and posted for all to see.

Acknowledging that you're human and get pissed off EVEN at the little loves of your life doesn't make you a bad mum. Having to walk away in order to calm down and catch your breath doesn't make you a bad mum. The next time you are knee-deep in regret or shame over the way you responded to your kids, rather than beat yourself up, try speaking to yourself kindly. With love – total and unconditional love.

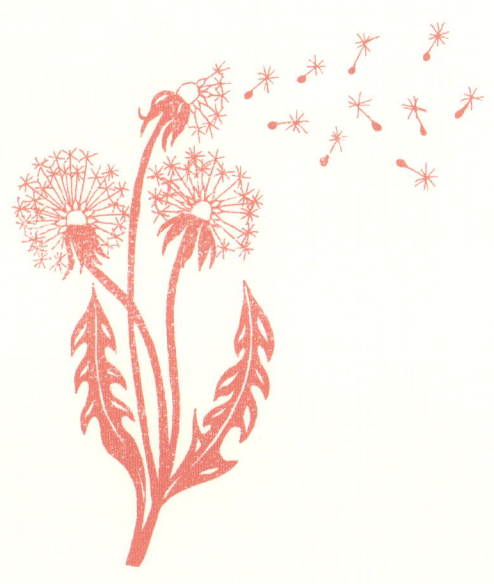

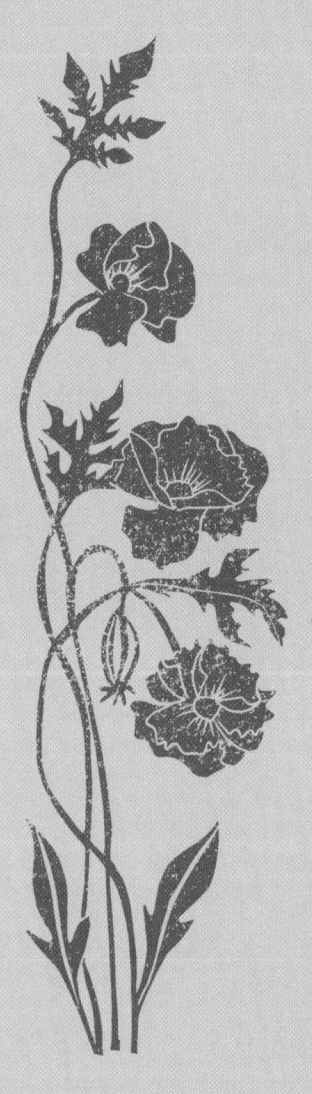

Have you considered all the things you are to your child?

When I comfort my children, I watch them as they melt into the safety of my body. When I get a phone call from school, I go to collect them and I see them sitting there with a quivering lip and tear-filled eyes but still holding it together. Until they see me.

When they see me, the tears fall and the sobs break free. Their mother is here. They are safe now. That's what I am for them. I am their place of safety and love, I am where they go when they need to be reminded of all that they are right now and all that they will be.

It is to me they run when they are hurt and scared. It is to me they turn when they are unsure of what to do or say next. It is to me they show their perfect 'special' stone that they're so proud of. It is to me they bring their rage and their darkest moments, secure in the knowledge that I am strong enough to withstand the storm.

This never changed for me, no matter how old I became. When I was happy, I called my mother. When I was down, I called my mother. She answered the phone and her voice soothed me like nothing else ever had or ever will. I felt the rhythm and cadence of her voice in every part of my being. Perhaps my body and soul remembered it from when she carried me.

I have called her many times with the intention of pretending everything was fine, only to hear her say 'Hello' and, with that one word, the tears fell and sobs broke free, just as sometimes happens with my children when they see me. She is still my place of safety in this world.

When I whisper words of love and encouragement to my children, I do so in the knowledge that my voice is one they will carry within themselves forever. It is a voice like no other. It is the voice of you, their mother.

Do you think there is a difference in sharing wisdom and offering a warning?

I saw a beautiful film clip where a mother was lying on the ground with her baby. The sun was shining and peeking through the gaps of the tree they were lying under. The mother was sharing that she felt like her life had just begun, that motherhood had given her true purpose, and she had found who she really was as a result of motherhood. She couldn't understand why so many seemed to offer harsh warnings about what it would be like to be a mother.

My heart sank with the words she spoke. Becoming a mother changed the direction of my life. And yet, for me, motherhood is as much an ending as it is a beginning. It can bring about the destruction of all that you were in order for you to become this version of yourself that exists today. And this can be hard.

As for purpose – well, what is purpose? Is it our search for self? Our hunger to feel like we are making a contribution to this world? Is it about the knowing of self? I imagine it is all of these things and much more. Motherhood has also shown me the role that purpose has played in helping me to become clearer about who I am. Perhaps this is my purpose in this lifetime – to know myself so well that other people's opinions of who I am, and who I am not, stays firmly within the realm of 'not my business'.

My babies introduced me to a love that literally takes my breath away at times. Perhaps I am naive to think that there is nothing like a mother's love, but this has been my experience both as a daughter and now as a mother.

People may 'warn' you about becoming a mother, but perhaps it comes from women who want to reassure you that although there is some danger ahead, you should not be afraid if you encounter murky parts of motherhood that you were not expecting. The danger lies not in the love you have for your baby – for that will most likely be pure and sacred – but in the fact that honest conversations about motherhood are often misconstrued as ungrateful complaints from unhappy mothers.

Dearest mothers, let's not shy away from sharing our beautiful highlights. It's wonderful to see mothers living the parts of their lives they show us with such happiness. Seeing them brings happy tears to my eyes as I remember the weight of my children when they were babies.

And please don't forget that perhaps what one person sees as a warning could in fact be wisdom being passed from one woman to another.

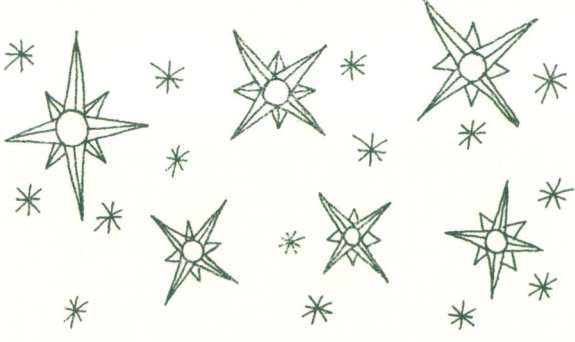

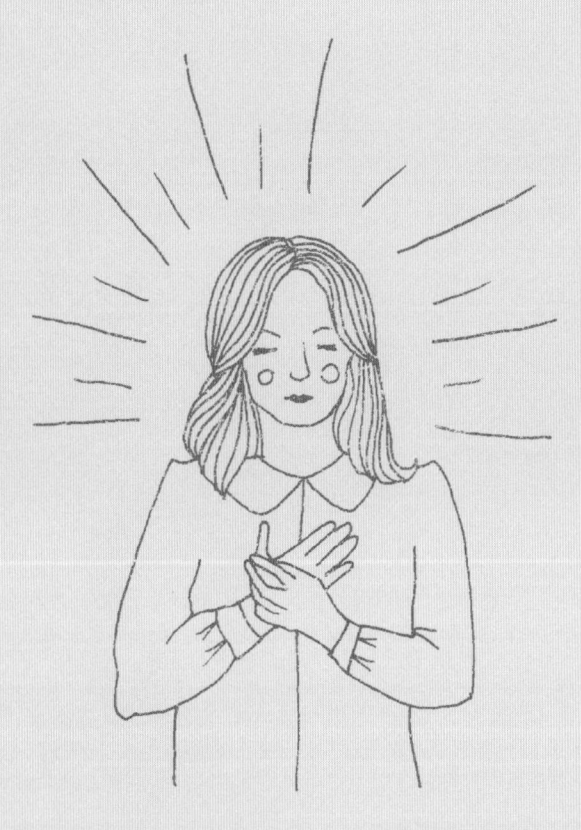

Are you the heartbeat of your home?

I heard a woman describe her mother as 'the heartbeat of the home'. My breath caught in my throat as I felt my own heart stutter at the truth of these words. My mother was the pulse of my childhood home. At times it was thundering and furious, and at other times strong and steady as it lulled me in safety and love. Am I the heartbeat of my home? Do I want that responsibility? Do I have a choice?

Sometimes it feels like a heavy burden but it is one that I would choose to carry over and over again if I had to. It is a beautiful burden to have. I look at my children and I offer myself to them. All of me is theirs to keep forever and ever. There are days when they get the parts of me that I would rather stay hidden but they hold me with love nonetheless.

There is not a part of me that does not sing with love for them. And yet my heart cannot live outside my body. It is vital for me in my life, and for my existence. Parts of it are mine and mine alone, to beat rhythmically and gloriously to my own tune.

Is this yet another paradox of motherhood? One that has me wanting to keep a sliver of what is mine for myself at the same time as offering it up to the most precious things that I have had the privilege of knowing.

On the days that I feel like maybe it's too much, and that maybe I am not doing a good job at this mothering beast, I close my eyes and put my hand on my chest. I listen to the beating of my heart. The one that beats for me and for them. *Mo chuisle* (my heartbeat).

If my children grow up and think of me as the heartbeat of their home, I hope they will remember the mother love that in turn fuelled me.

What does silence sound like?

There are times when I really listen to my children quietening down at bedtime. I love to pay attention to how they start off so excited and full of chat when they first go to bed. There are squeals of laughter and loud thumps as they jump off beds. I hear toys and books being strewn about the floor and serious discussions being had, the details of which my adult mind cannot fully comprehend but I know are important nonetheless.

If I wasn't paying attention, I might not notice that the noise level drops a little and the squeals quieten to bursts of conversation every now and again. I only notice because tonight is one of those nights where my attention wanders from what I am working on to what is going on upstairs. There is still the odd bang here and there. Perhaps a teddy has been thrown or a toy has fallen off the bed, its service no longer required for the night. Time passes and the silence grows.

I sit in the kitchen working away but I can hear that sleep is calling for my children. There are no more loud noises, only the occasional quietly spoken sentence passed between them as they begin to be lulled into slumber. And then there are no more words. I feel the silence descend like a cloak upon the house.

After a while, I make my way upstairs and look in on them. I soak in the details of how each of them likes to sleep – details that I will one day joke with them about. I see Barbie's feet peeking out of Molly's quilt and Fionn is curled up on his side, his precious Pokémon cards tucked safely under his pillow. Their little bodies have succumbed to rest and they are quiet for the first time since they opened their eyes this morning.

It has been a long day.

There is something so very special and sacred about this silence. I can feel it, it's filled with unconditional love and forgiveness for those tense moments that occur over the course of the day. I take my fill of the silence, and allow it to work its magic as I look at my children sleeping.

The sound of silence can be so healing and rejuvenating to a mother's heart.

What soothes your mother heart?

I think a mother's heart opens at night. I think it opens in order to soothe and tend to her bruised mind and soul. As her heart opens, it fills her with thoughts and images and feelings of love so that her frustrations and disappointments and rages of the day begin to dissolve.

Guilt may linger, but the sting is taken out of it when she sees them safe and so very, very loved, tucked in their beds and snoring softly with the well-earned exhaustion that comes from a hard day's play.

She has done her best for another day.

It's almost as though we are called to stand over them at night, to spend time just looking at them and listening to the sound of their breathing. In those precious night-time moments, there are no demands being placed, no questions to be answered, no fights to be broken up – we can just soak them in.

When I'm in their room gently fixing their blankets and quietly emptying their beds of toys, it feels like I have entered a sacred space filled with hope and tenderness and a love so strong that at times it can feel too big for one mother to carry. On the other side of this great love is fear – fear for what we cannot control. It's a fine line to walk and at times I dwell on the scary side for longer than I would like.

But let us not dwell on what we cannot control, my friend, not tonight. Let us breathe in their beauty for they will not be this little for long.

What tiny moments have faded from memory, but live on in you?

I can't be the only one who loves going through old photos. I look at ones from when my boy was a baby and it feels like a lifetime ago. I remember thinking at the time that I would NEVER forget how it felt to hold the weight of him in my arms as he snuggled in and drifted off to sleep while staring back at me, seeing straight into my soul.

But I have forgotten.

I frantically try to pull up a memory of watching him fall asleep but all I get is image upon image of my eight-year-old boy laughing as he burrows down under his quilt, using everything he's got to bargain for more time to read.

I suppose this is the way of it. To live in the present with him and soak in all of his beautiful, fleeting boyishness, my head has to let go of older moments in order to make way for the new. But my heart will never forget. That I know with certainty.

I might not be able to recall the exact tone of his snorting laughter or the heaviness of his breath that would confirm he was finally asleep, but the minute I see a photo of him from his baby days, my heart explodes with such love and knowing that it reassures me.

This body of mine that carried him will never forget. We are so woven together that there is no need to worry about forgetting. Our bodies remember even when our memories fade.

What have you taken for granted but now treasure?

Oh my boy, I didn't notice when you stopped being that plump, curly-haired baby. You're eight now, the chubbiness is long gone and so are the blonde curls. Oh my heart . . .

Fionn and I went to the shops together last Sunday, just the two of us. He insisted on coming with me and I was immediately suspicious that he wanted a toy or something else that he would be asking me for. He doesn't usually want to go places with me – his dad is his number one.

We got to the first shop and picked up what we needed. All the while he was running around the place, picking up one Christmas decoration after another.

'Mam, look at this. I love penguins. Do you think they get cold?'

'Put it down Fionn, come on, let's keep going. We need to get some other stuff from the next shop.'

I'm always hurrying, always trying to get somewhere.

We got to the next shop, I automatically reached my hand out for his and he took it. When he slid his hand into mine, I immediately realized that it had been a long time since I had held the weight of my boy's hand in mine. My heart exploded in my chest and I stopped dead in the shop and looked at him.

This beautiful boy of mine. I wondered when we stopped holding hands. Maybe it's because his sister is usually with us and she always holds my hand while he, my little ball of energy, runs and jumps and hops around the place.

I stared at him with tears in my eyes.

'It's been a long time since we've held hands.'

'I know, Mama.' He started to take his hand out of mine and I asked him if we could hold hands for a little longer. I told him that I loved the feeling of his hand in mine, and that I had missed that feeling. He smiled, said 'yes' and off we walked for a moment, hand in hand. He quickly got over the hand-holding and tore off around the shop. I haven't got over the hand-holding as quickly. The feeling lingers in me still. The feel of his fingers is so different now – his hand was warm and dry, and no longer the clammy, pudgy one of before.

For almost the first two years of his life, he and I were always together. Where I went, he went. We cuddled and we played, and rolled around the floor together. He climbed all over me for fun and burrowed into me for safety and love. I have thousands of photos documenting our days together, and for days after the hand-holding, I pored over all those photos again.

I didn't notice those days disappearing. We never do. They were hard days – and lonely. They were intense and exhausting as it was mainly just him and me during the days. I could never have imagined a time when I would stop dead in my tracks because I suddenly realized I hadn't held my son's hand in a long time.

What once I took for granted, I now treasure.

May I always know the weight of my boy's hand in mine.

What do you think your children learn from watching you?

I often wonder what my daughter will remember the most about me. I wonder what she'll blame me for and what she'll say that her mother taught her.

I sometimes forget that it's not just me who learns from the events in my life. My daughter is watching me. She's learning how to operate in this world, and how to speak out and stand up for herself, from me. She's learning that it's ok to tell someone that she doesn't want to be kissed, picked-up, cuddled, tickled or touched.

I'm trying to teach her that she isn't responsible for other people and their behaviour. If someone pretends to cry because she won't kiss them, I tell her that it's ok. Their response to her doesn't mean she has to now do what she said she didn't want to do, just because someone doesn't like or agree with her decision.

I hope the roots that we're nurturing in her will run so strong and deep that they will keep her grounded in her worth when she's old enough to understand just how precious her belief in herself is. One thing I've learned for sure over these last few years of motherhood is that our children are wise beyond their years. They KNOW when our words don't match our actions, and when we are not honouring the very lesson we are preaching to them.

They do what we do, not what we say.

The older she gets, the more she sees. The more she sees, the more she does. The more she does, the more she starts to cement the foundations of her future. I want that foundation to be rock-solid. If someone tells her she has failed, if she questions who she is or her place in the world, or if she finds herself pushed to a point she fears she may never return from, I want her to remember that she is the one who will dictate her greatness, and no one else.

I want her to remember that she ALWAYS has a choice.

I want her to know that she doesn't need to wait for someone else to see her greatness. Waiting is a waste of time.

I hope she will remember that I don't apologize for prioritizing my needs. I want her to know that she won't need to either.

I want her to know that if she wants a seat at the table, she must go and take it. For she is worthy of it all.

I want her to remember that she ALWAYS has a choice.

She's just . . .
How significant is the role of a mother?

She's just trying for a baby. She's just pregnant. She's just having her first scan and hearing her baby's heartbeat for the first time. She's just excited because she's a first-time mum. She's just finding pregnancy difficult. She's just not feeling herself as she figures out how to move forward with this new version of herself. She's just tired. She's just heavily pregnant. She's just in labour. She's just being induced.

She's just feeling traumatized. She's just had a baby and she's now just feeding that baby. She's just trying to stick with the breastfeeding even though her nipples are bleeding and sore. She's just exhausted. She's just trying to survive on tiny amounts of broken sleep. She's just a bit sore from her stitches, which makes it difficult for her to sit up in bed at night to feed. She's just feeling a bit down. She's just wanting a good cry but doesn't want people to think she's not coping.

She's just getting used to things. She's just upset that her partner doesn't seem to be doing as badly as her at this parenting thing. She's just so exhausted she no longer knows what day it is. She's just fed up with people telling her what she should and shouldn't do. She's just so happy to be here with her baby.

She's just so busy she has no time for herself. She's just making the breakfast, the lunch and then it's time for dinner. She's just tidying up and changing the beds.

She's just answering the 75,089th question of the day. She's just going to the shop. She's just sitting on the couch, holding her entire universe in her arms because they are upset and no one else but her will do. She's just lying on the floor, willing herself not to scream if she hears 'Mama' one more time. She's just lying awake all night because her baby isn't well. She's just feeling a bit lost. She's just wondering if other mums feel like this. She's just getting on with it. She's just doing what she does best.

She's just a mum.
Oceans are not 'just' oceans.
Stars are not 'just' stars.
You are not 'just' a mum.
You are someone's entire world.
You are their mother.
You are their mother.

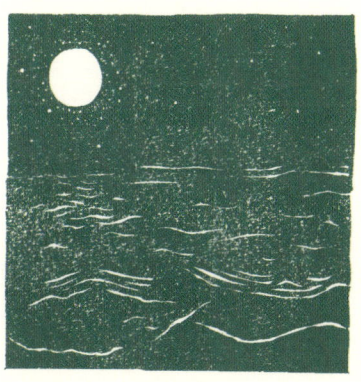

Are you a great mum?

We've all been there – we've all questioned if we really have what it takes to be a great mum. We look around us and cannot help but fall into the giant sinkhole of never-ending doom and gloom that's more commonly known as 'The Comparison Trap'. Before we know it, we're comparing who has the grimmest feet and hairiest toes (you'd definitely win). Well, fear not. My years of study and extensive research have provided me with pure scientific gold. I am confident that this data is solid and the type of testing that was undertaken can be done the world over and still produce the same results.

Are you ready to discover the 'Top Ten Signs To Look For To Know If You Are A Great Mum'? Ok, let's dive in.

1. Do you have kids? You're a GREAT mum.
2. Do you sometimes want to run from your house screaming and never come back? If the answer is 'Yes' (I'm laughing at the fact that I said 'IF') you're a GREAT mum.
3. Are you tired to the bone of hearing someone (by 'someone', obviously I mean your kids) shouting at the top of their lungs for you to come and clean their bum after doing a poo? FOR THE LOVE OF GOD . . . WHEN WILL THIS STOP? Still a GREAT mum.
4. When you pick up a small mirror and breathe on it, does it steam up with your breath? You're a GREAT mum.
5. I moustache you a question: The last time you happened to glance at your upper lip in the mirror of the visor, in your car, in the unforgiving, cruel and harsh light of sunshine, what did you see? A GREAT mum.

6. Are you familiar with the feeling of wanting time to stand still so that you can soak yourself in the feel of the weight of your baby? So that you can etch into your heart the rhythm of your child's breathing when they lie there asleep in their bed, quiet for what feels like the first time since they opened their eyes in the morning? GREAT mum.
7. Have you ever felt so lost that you quietly questioned (to yourself, of course. Imagine the shame if you were to talk openly about how you felt?) your purpose here in this lifetime? Is this it? Is this what the rest of my life is going to look like? Not knowing who I am anymore? Guess what . . . You're a GREAT mum.
8. Have you ever woken yourself up farting? (asking for a friend). GREAT Mum.
9. Are you the woman who questions her worth and what she brings to the table? Do you find yourself weary from wondering if you're enough? If you are and you do, please trust me when I say that you are enough, you are loved, you are worthy of it all and you are a GREAT mum.
10. Do you ever have heart-bursting moments of complete clarity where you get a glimpse of how crucial and fundamental and life-changing what you do actually is? That's because YOU ARE A GREAT MUM.

Therefore, in conclusion, to sum it all up . . . from one great mum to another, I see you.

What is a mother?

My eyes and my heart have been opened to the spectrum of mothering that exists beyond what I have always known.

A mother to me was softness and strictness. When I was young, my mother was not my friend – she was very much my MOTHER. She was rules and housekeeping, she was pocket-money, pick-ups and drop offs. She was relentless in her dedication to making sure my brother and I got to where we needed to be.

My mother was the cushion I landed on after hitting the wall of her firmly held boundary. She was my constant, and one I took for granted as is the way of all children. And that's ok, this is the way of it. My children do the same. They are so free to revolt against me because I work so hard to lay the foundation of unconditional love and security on which they build their frequent uprisings. One day, when they are older, they too will see the price that was paid for their freedom of expression. It is a price we all pay, painfully but usually willingly.

What is a mother? A mother is someone who watches from the sidelines and holds themselves back to let you fall so that you learn to pick yourself back up again. A mother is the person who tells you that to get better at it, you have to do it yourself. A mother is someone who believes that the world is a better place with you in it, and spends the rest of their life reminding you of how significant and important and loved you are.

A mother is someone who believes in you – *really* believes in the very essence of all that you are. A mother sees through your bravado and bullshit, and loves you in ALL of your glory. In my case my mother answered the phone and knew to stay silent while I tried to breathe my way through the pain of what I so desperately wanted to say but had no words for. In this silence I found the solace that I sought. In that moment, there was only me and my mother. Forever.

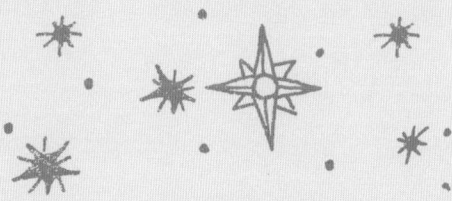

There is no **perfect**,
no ideal standard.
There is only **you** and
the love that you have for
those you mother.
Isn't that
wonderful?

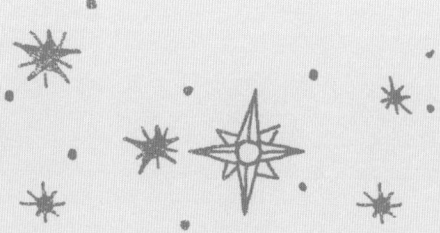

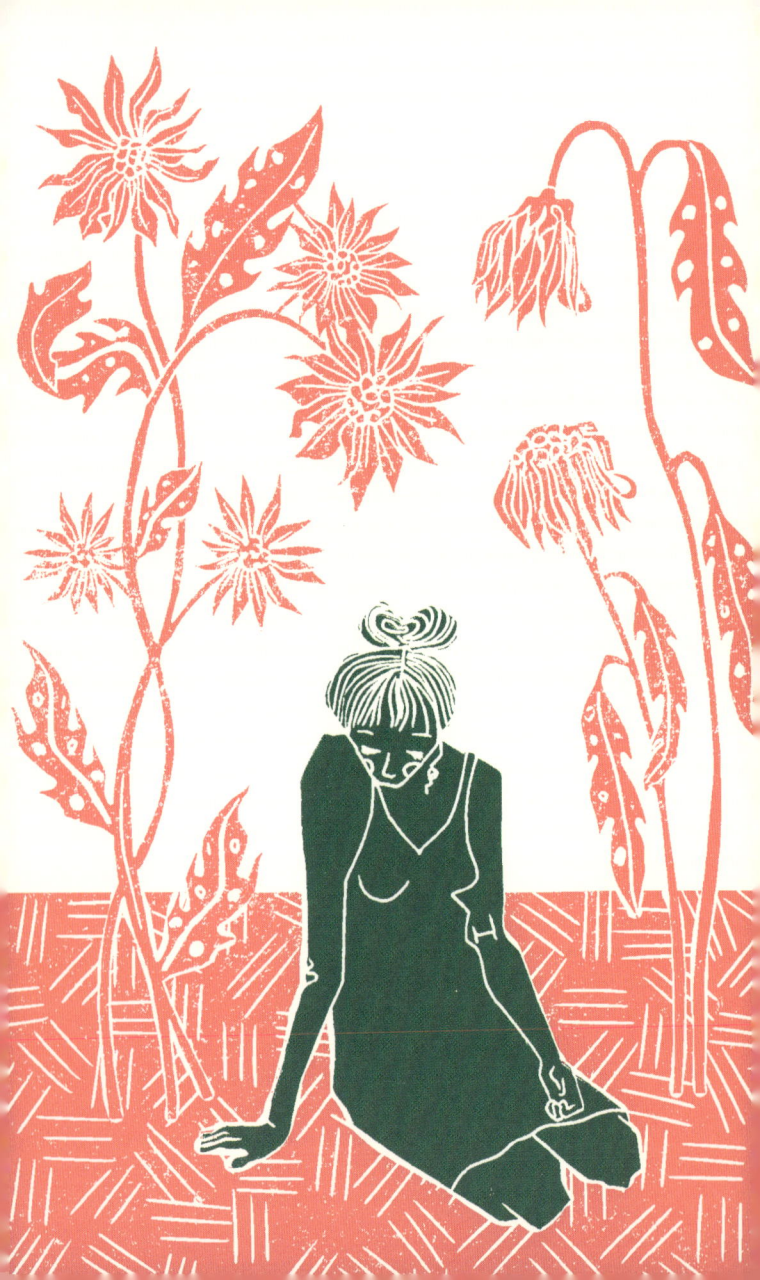

The grief of a mother

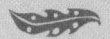

When I became a mother, I felt lost in the magnitude and intensity of love, loss, pain, fear, excitement and hope. When my mother died, I felt so lost, for all the same reasons. I feel like I can speak quite confidently about what it feels like to be lost.

However, I'm starting to believe we are never lost. I believe we find ourselves in the places of our lives that our hearts and minds have tried to shield us from. We know that 'stuff' happens but we convince ourselves that somehow it happens to 'other' people and not us. No one who I have encountered enters into motherhood truly believing that they will be the unlucky one with post-natal depression, a fourth-degree tear from childbirth, a sick baby, incontinence, a relationship that breaks down, a never-ending feeling of guilt and overwhelm, a loss of identity . . . [insert your own description here].

All of these things, though, can, and do, happen. All you have to do is go online and search for these topics, or go and talk to other mums and you will see just how common all of the above actually are. But somehow we enter into motherhood for the first time believing that *everything will be grand*. We'll be grand. Motherhood will be grand.

We do this in the rest of our lives too. Some of us walk through it, untouched for a long time by the hard stuff; others are barely out of the womb when their challenges start. It's hard and it hurts. It's beautiful and it brings me so much joy. It's life.

What I've discovered in the last few years is that community will help you through the toughest of times. To know that you are not alone in how you feel is life-saving. To speak to those who have walked this path before you is so comforting, and heartbreakingly sad at the same time. It's only then that you see the dim glow of the lights they've left behind them so that those who follow can find their way in the darkness.

Walking with grief, like most of the transformational experiences in life, is something that is unique and personal to us all (and loss doesn't need to mean the death of a loved one – it can be applied to so much more). Only I can work my way through this but that doesn't mean I have to walk alone. I am grateful for those who walk beside me, even if it's just to hold my hand for a second, or to catch my eye and share a smile and a heartbeat together.

And so now I too will leave a light on.

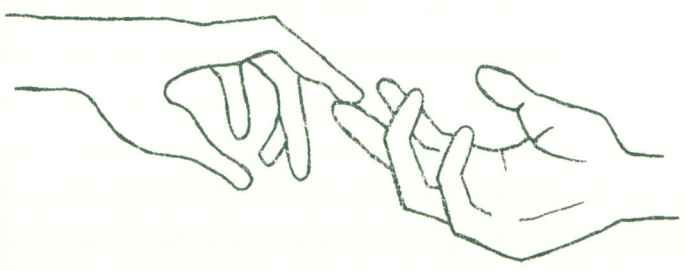

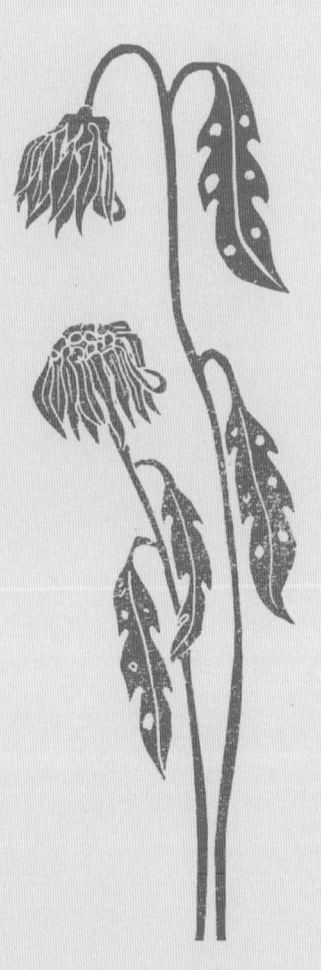

Have you ever stood in the place where grief lives?

There is a sacredness to holding the gaze of those who have felt the loss of a loved one (for me, the loss of my mother). There is no need for words; our hearts search and connect, they beat to the rhythm of a similar drum. There is an honouring. An ease. A space in which we each find it easier to exhale because we are in the company of someone who needs no false platitudes of how well we're doing even though we may be weeping on the inside. We see each other's pain and respect it. It is a privilege to hear someone speak the name of those they've lost.

I can tell you that this place I'm in, this place I never imagined being at this stage of my life, is a curious place to inhabit and call home. Yet even in the darkest and heaviest of moments, the ones that seem to descend like an invisible and relentless pressure, there is still light and there is still love.

Every breath I take reminds me of the privilege of being here. There have been times when I have gasped on my inhale as I felt like I was suffocating in this new reality where my mother no longer lives. And then my exhale comes along. It reminds me. It teaches me that there are bigger things than us at play here. My breath releases with ease, I am no longer fearful. But I am still heartbroken. And perhaps you know that.

And I am painfully grateful for those I meet who stand with me in the places where grief resides, for this is a place where many fear to tread.

What makes you feel alive?

I've been thinking a lot about my new love of sea-swimming. I feel like I am answering an unspoken call each time I make my way towards the sea. It makes me feel alive. Yes, perhaps this is why I love it so much.

When I break communion with the waves, I am forced to think of nothing but my breath. I hear it rushing out of my body as my lungs fight to claw it back in. As I drop down into the water I at once feel part of it and connected to myself and my own life again.

I like to watch the sky as it moves above me and I feel my mother's presence. It is in these moments that I feel close to her. I love the horizon, and the magical place where the sea kisses the sky. I believe that if the sea can do this, then so too can I. I stare at the meeting place of heaven and earth and then close my eyes so I can meet her there for a moment. The sea bears witness to my tears – it welcomes them home as its own. Salt water to salt water.

Sometimes my children come with me when I swim. They play on the shoreline and I watch them. It is at these moments, with the horizon at my back and my children at my front that I am filled with both gratitude and sorrow. I am humbled by the gifts of life and love.

And so today I will swim to celebrate my mother, one of the greatest loves of my life.

I like to watch

the sky as it moves

above me and I feel my

mother's
presence.

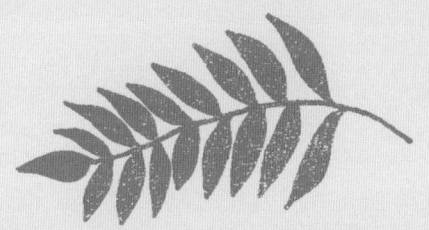

Aren't words **powerful?** They are our **legacy**, and they will linger in the **hearts** and **minds** of our **children** long after we are gone.

What words connect you?

'I love you more.'

My mother and I started saying this to each other a few years ago. We were rounding off one of our many daily text chats and I told her I loved her. She immediately replied, 'I love you more'. I said that wasn't true – there was no way she could possibly love me more than I loved her, and there was no body or heart big enough for more love than what I carried within me for her.

This sentence was eventually shortened to 'you more' and we would randomly message each other with just those two words. Aren't words powerful? They are our legacy, and they will linger in the hearts and minds of our children long after we are gone.

It's not just the words, it's the person and the special, private meaning that lies behind them. I hear her voice when I read these words and I imagine her face as she typed them; she would be smiling. These words build a picture in my mind. They remind me to savour the fleeting moments of bliss and joy and love and hope and comfort, for they are never guaranteed and, in time, they will become nothing but memories to last a lifetime, and these memories will help soothe but not fix a broken heart.

Of course she loved me more, we both knew it. How could she not? She was my mother, and I know what a mother's love feels like.

It is a love like no other. It is as terrifying as it is beautiful. There are times when I look at my children and I feel the weight of the world when I imagine what their lives will be like. Will they be healthy? Will they be happy? Am I giving them everything they need in order to take flight when they are ready? But I cannot live like that – we are not meant to stay suspended in fear. We must trust that life is life and we don't get to tip-toe through it without it costing us greatly.

Have you ever thought about all the thresholds you've crossed in your life?

On Monday, 6 August 2012, I was sitting beside my mum and we were in the passenger seats of the van my dad was driving. We were heading into Glasgow so that me, my (new) husband Stuart and his family could fly back to Dublin.

The reason this memory stays so alive for me is because of the role that loss and grief play in my life. They visit me from time to time and they descend heavily into my mind and soul.

You see, I was a newly married woman. In fact, I had got married only three days before this journey into Glasgow and the weekend had been filled with such joy and love and laughter. I was buzzing from the high I was on and couldn't wait to get back to Dublin so that Stuart and I could head to New York the next day for our honeymoon. Life was good and I was indeed a happy bride.

We met Stuart, his mum, dad, sister and brother at the train station. They had taken a taxi from the hotel to the station and I had chosen to go in the van with my mum and dad.

As we all congregated in the bar at the train station, my mum and dad eventually stood to leave. I held eyes with my mum and I started to cry. This felt like such a monumental moment for us as daughter and parents. I was now a married woman and my mum and dad were leaving me with my brand new husband (who I had already been living with for many years). I felt confused as to why I felt so sad.

I didn't know at the time that I was grieving the crossing of a threshold. Deep within me I felt a sadness: I was no longer who I had been and yet parts of me will always hold the memories of the girl who grew up in Kipps Ave.

The thing about crossing thresholds – leaving a time or place in our lives – is that we don't usually know we are in the midst of it until later. Thresholds, endings and beginnings are not always clear until we have some distance between those moments and we can look back and see them for what they were. A loss. A moment in time where something ended and something new began. A gain.

Watching my parents leave that day struck something deep within me, and I felt tremendous sadness. My husband and his family all hugged me. I felt loved but that didn't change my feelings of loss. And that's ok.

I can feel grief and still be grateful for what I have. I can feel loss and still acknowledge what I have gained.

Loss doesn't need to mean the death of a loved one. It can be applied to so much more. There are a lifetime of moments like this one, moments that often go unacknowledged and yet sit within us like a soft ache when remembered. Exploring these memories helps me make sense of who I was, who I have become and who I am yet to be.

And so it is in motherhood. From being the mother of a newborn to standing at the side of a football pitch on a Sunday morning watching my ten-year-old son celebrate a goal.

There have been millions of tiny and monumental losses to get to where I am today.

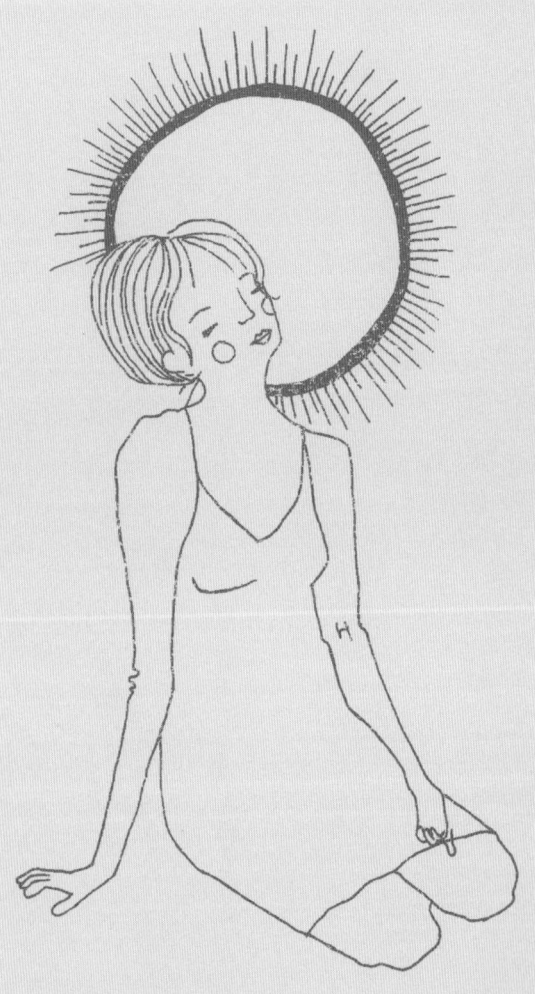

Do you find it painful to accept what is rather than what you think it should be?

When I think about who I have been and the realms of hell that I have visited, it causes me to catch my breath at the beauty that I still see in this world. We can be surrounded by and engulfed in darkness, choking on desperate hope. And then we may feel the sunlight on our faces again – and for a few seconds we know it feels magnificent, and it reminds us that we will be ok. In time.

I never imagined that I would lose my mother the way I did. To sit beside her as she drew her last breaths and send her on her way with words of love and gratitude that she was mine for a while is probably the most painful but beautiful moment of my life so far. I know what it feels like to be in the presence of love so pure that you feel no pain, only love for what is. Yes, that moment passes. It was never meant to last forever but the memory of it will stay with me until my own dying day.

Has hope ever let you down?

Has there ever been a time in your life where you couldn't eat, sleep or do anything other than hope and beg and pray for a resolution that you knew deep down wasn't possible? I have, and it has tainted my relationship with hope.

I remember hearing the line 'hope is a beggar' a few years ago. It didn't really make much sense to me at the time. I remember thinking it was a strange sentence, and one I easily laughed off. Yet it stayed with me. 'Hope is a beggar.' Every now and then I'd think of this sentence, still no clearer on what it actually meant. I then learned that it was said by Jim Carrey in a speech he made in 2014. Still made no sense really.

A year ago today was the point in my life when I finally understood what the line 'hope is a beggar' meant. The taste of hope in my mouth became rancid as I spoke with the doctor, desperately waiting to hear what I knew I would never hear.

It was late December when I was given a prescription for drugs that would 'help' my body to begin the process it was reluctant to do itself. The purpose of the drugs was to initiate the miscarriage that my body refused to accept had happened. My body would not accept what my heart knew to be true – my pregnancy was no more.

Hope curdled and solidified in my stomach. It turned poisonous and slowly made its way through my veins leaving me with nothing but a hollow emptiness keeping me alive. The very existence of hope seemed to taunt me in my desperation; I would have given anything for things to be different. I rode hope hard and it left me high and dry.

The drugs did their job. I went into the new year no longer a mum of two with one on the way. There were moments of pure and utter despair. How can this be? What good is hope when there is no hope? I have no answers for these questions, and I never will. I have had to choose to accept what it is rather than what I wanted it to be. And this has been one of the toughest lessons of my life. Hope deserved no place in my life,

I have yet to make my peace with hope. Maybe I never will – who says I have to be at peace with hope? Perhaps it is a lifelong relationship that will ebb and flow.

In the speech that Jim Carrey gives, he says: 'Not hope but faith. I don't believe in hope. Hope is a beggar. Hope walks through fire. Faith leaps over it.' And I get that now, all of it.

In the absence of hope I have faith. Faith in myself and this painful but magnificent thing I call my life.

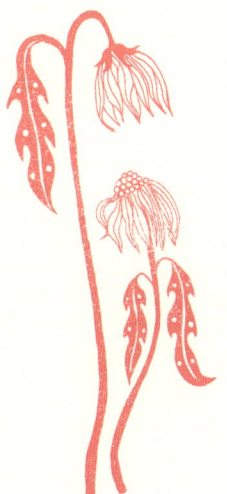

Are there parts of your life where you play it safe?

In becoming a mother, I lost parts of my soul that I will spend the rest of my life searching for. This is the price I paid. In losing my mother, I also lost parts of my soul. The absence of her is felt in every waking moment. I am learning that this hurt and pain is an honouring of this life I live.

Perhaps these parts of my soul had to leave in order for me to survive, and to have a chance at becoming who I need to be. I have learned harsh and beautiful lessons. I have been brought to my knees many times. I have outgrown old ways of thinking and been humbled by people and circumstances. I have roared and wept with pain that I will carry with me to the grave. I have laughed and rejoiced with joy and love too many times to count. I have lived.

I will search for the missing parts of my soul forever. I know they call to me. They lie in wait, ready to be reclaimed when I am able to do so. I wonder who I will become in the reintegration process. Parts of my soul travel this earth – they roam free and wild. They wait for me to find my way back to them. And so I forge ahead. I open my arms and my heart to all that lies here with me in this darkness of grief and sorrow. These events changed me. They ripped out from under me who I thought I was and showed me that I could choose to cling on to a version of myself that wasn't real or I could embrace the inevitability of who I could be.

My heart has cracked, shattered and broken. I have spent time picking shards of it off the floor, desperate to piece it back together, and make it what it was before. What I didn't realize is that our hearts have to break. They have shells around them that shatter and crack and fall apart as we go through life. Underneath all these shells that we mistakenly think of as our hearts, lies the real thing. It beats powerfully under these protective casings. It gets stronger and bigger with every pounding it takes.

You can try and protect your heart – the path of safety is there should you wish to take it, but I have learned this too has a price to pay. You can spend your life trying to keep your heart safe but in doing so you will rob yourself of living.

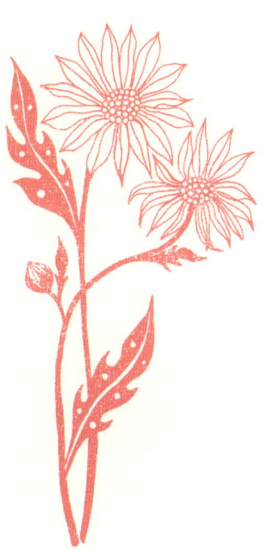

Some days we **survive** with strength, other days we **barely** get through.

Have you ever found yourself on your knees in the ashes of your life?

Sometimes we don't rise powerfully from the ashes. Sometimes we kneel there in the middle of them, wounded and bleeding, torn to shreds from what we've been through, confused as to how we got here and uncertain of where to go next.

Experiences – the ones that rip through our lives and leave us silently screaming in pain – sear themselves into our souls. They become as much a part of us as the air we breathe. They are what makes us who we are, and when we look back through the healing passage of time, we will see that these moments have helped define the women we will one day become.

Some days we survive with strength. Other days we barely get through. Keep breathing, knowing that soon the day will come when it's no longer painful to do so.

There is an inevitable surrender to the full kaleidoscope of life, eventually. Eventually.

But know that when you are kneeling there, feeling exposed and unsure, in the ashes and remnants of the person you were before this experience touched your life, you are on the verge of a becoming.

Picking up the tiny slivers of faith and courage may very well be what will get you through these days, and that's ok. There is time for you to rise, my friend. There is time.

Perhaps what you need right now is to run your fingers through the ashes of what has been, lie down among the remnants of who you used to be and breathe in her essence. She is no longer who you are. Take courage from her and know that you have everything you need right now in order to stand again.

There are many ways to get back on your feet, none of them better than any other. Go slowly and with grace, my friend.

Do you believe in magic?

I believe the whispers of love from our mothers linger in us and run through our veins.

I tiptoe quietly into the shared bedroom of my children – Molly is to the right and Fionn is to the left. As I stand between their two beds, I feel fierce and fragile at the same time. I listen to the rhythm of their breathing and I close my eyes. I want my other senses to kick in so that I feel connected to my children with every fibre of my being. My heart tightens with joy and a kind of sorrow when I think about the lives they have ahead of them. I feel a beautiful sadness when I look at their long limbs and freckly noses. They are babies no more.

I soak in every inch of Moll as I rearrange the quilt that she has wrapped herself up in. I look at her in awe. I wonder how it's possible that she is mine for a while. I watch her chest rise and fall, and I kiss her goodnight and whisper in her ear how much I love her. I know her soul hears me, and harnesses my love and stores it for the days when she will need it most.

I turn around and look at my son. He sleeps so soundly. His blanket is twisted around his body and I take great care as I untangle him from it. I could watch him all night. A painful ease comes over me when I indulge in these moments of stillness with my boy. From the moment he opens his eyes, there is an intensity and noise that surrounds him. It is such a privilege to see him rest, to see him so at peace. I call upon my mothering magic and I whisper in his ear. I remind him of how loved he is and how loved he will always be. I kiss him goodnight.

As I stand to leave, I feel the whispers of love from my own mother pulse through my veins. These are the days my soul has been preparing for. These are the days when I need her love the most.

The magic of a mother is real.

The **magic** of a
mother
is **real**.

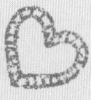

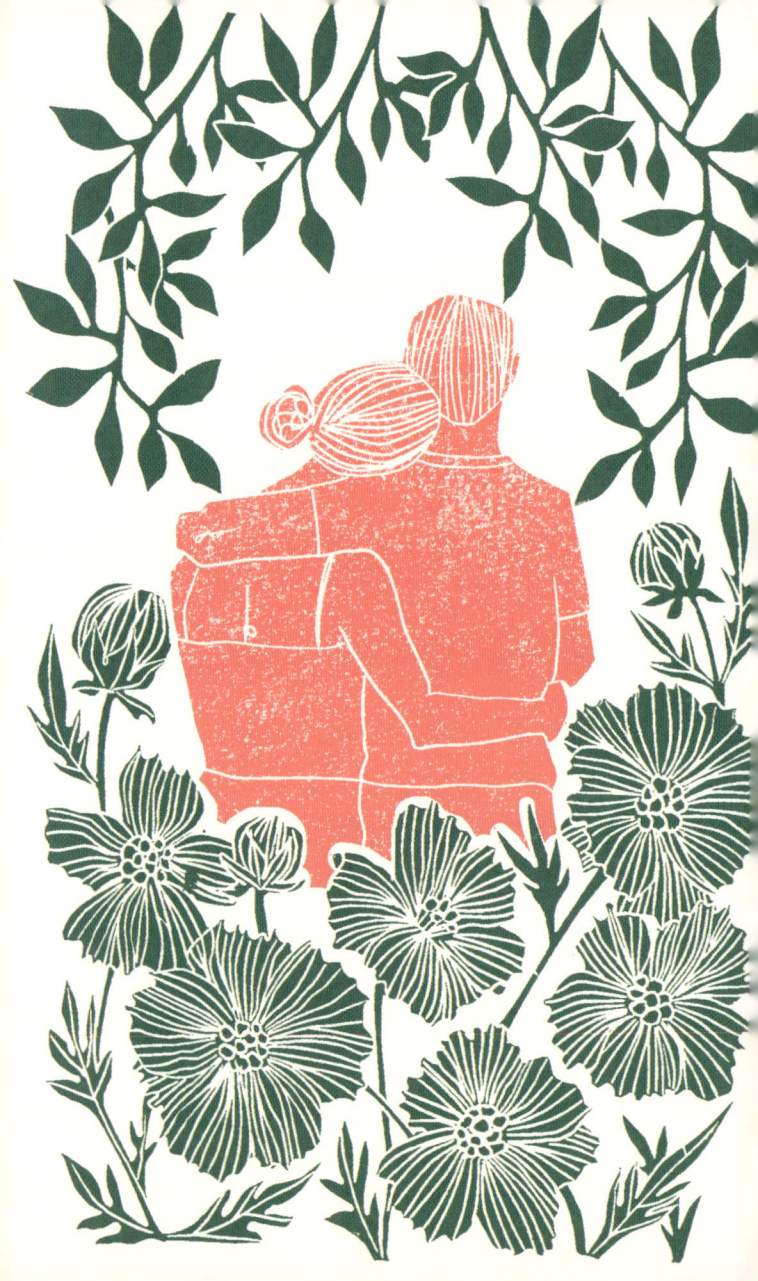

A mother
and her
loved ones

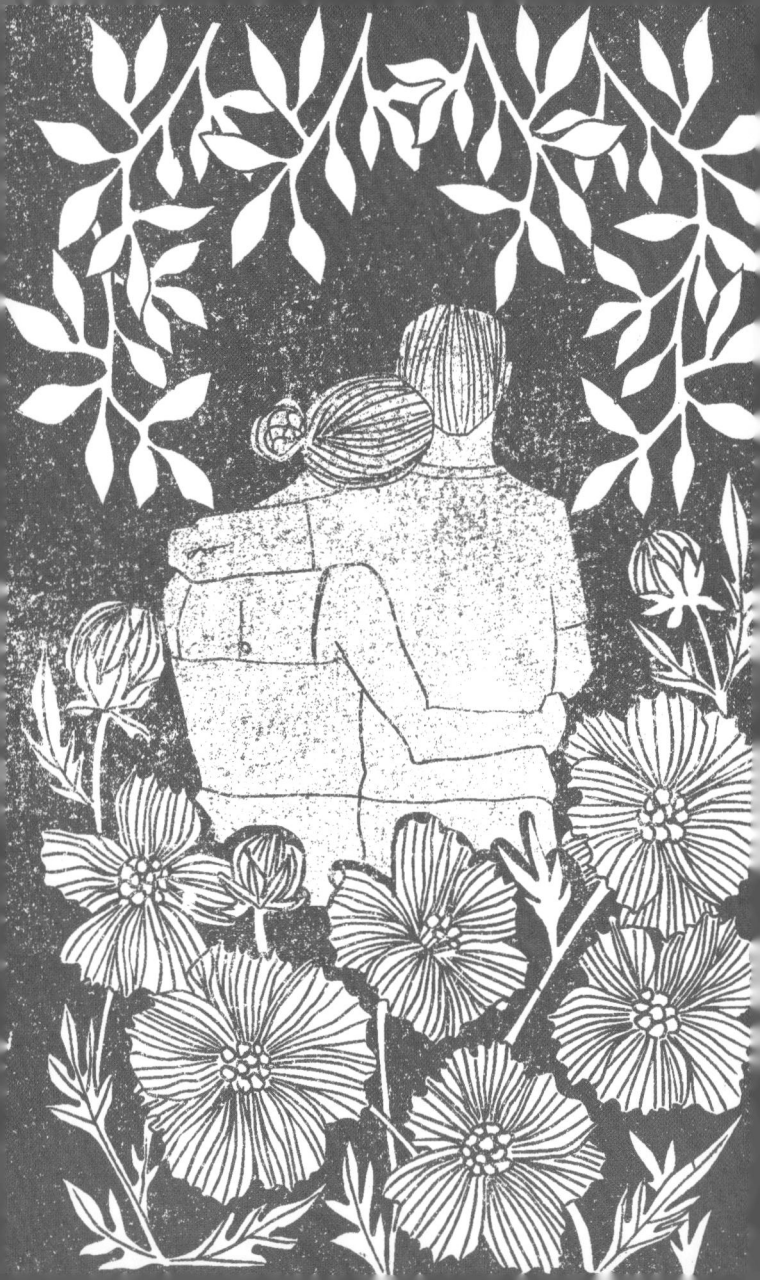

There's a slow seduction into servantry for the partner who has become the stay-at-home parent. As we take on more responsibility for the cleaning, the cooking and the organizing of the baby clothes, we set up patterns that will inevitably lead to resentment down the line at the disproportionate burden of domestic responsibility.

Having my children bear witness to me becoming the idealized self-appointed sacrificial lamb for my family is not an option for me. It is my intention that I will not taint their childhood with the discomfort of witnessing their mother running herself into the ground in an attempt to live up to standards of motherhood that serve the many while neglecting the woman. I cannot bear the thought of them discussing me when they are older and talking about how bad they feel at the fact their mother sacrificed herself and her dreams for them. My dreams and ambitions (or lack thereof) are not their responsibilities to carry. Furthermore, I will not burden my children with the lies that their mother had no needs, or that their mother was a selfless woman.

When the time comes and my children are off living their lives, I hope they will remember that their parents, their mother, showed them that there was nothing shameful or bad about chasing their dreams. I would rather they reminisce over the times we all discussed our dreams together instead of them looking back and wondering why their mother stayed silent when it came to her own life. What I do and say now impacts what they believe is possible for themselves in the future. And this is why I include myself, my dreams, my failures and my ambitions in the conversations we have. This is why I keep choosing to let them witness me in all of my imperfect humanity, for it is this that makes me the mother I am.

Do you want your loved ones to be happy?

When we think about how we want our loved ones to be, we want them full of life, interested in things, and to have hobbies. We want them to be passionate and animated about something, and excited for something. We want to hear them speak about a subject that makes their faces light up and their voice change pitch because they're so alive, and so full of passion, when talking about it. We want them to be happy and fulfilled.

Why, then, do we find it so difficult to say we want that for ourselves too?

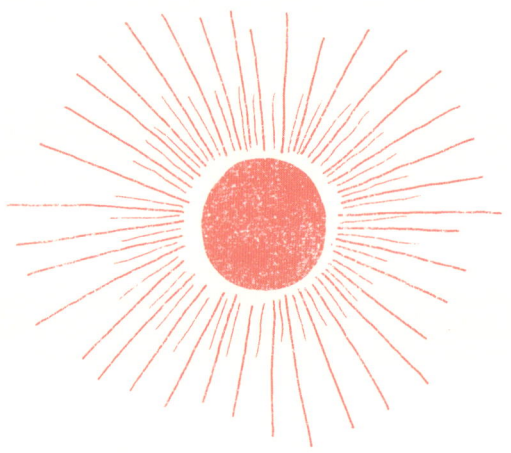

Can you hold several things to be true at the same time?

Can you love motherhood and
still want something outside of it for yourself?
Can you be so in love with the people in your life but
still want more for yourself?
Can you want to burst with happiness and still want to cry
because there's sorrow inside of you?
Can you feel utterly content and be bored out of your mind
with the monotony of motherhood?
Can you look around and be so grateful for the life you have
and the people in it, but still know with certainty that there
is more to come?
Can you feel trapped and also know you are exactly where
you are meant to be?
Can you feel it all, every last breath, laugh, touch of the
hand, intimate gaze and still feel numb?
Can you crave attention but want to retreat to the stillness
of your darkened room?
Can you long, with every fibre of your being, for time to
stand still and yet still count down every second to bedtime?
Can you hope for a better day tomorrow but still trust that
today has not been a failure?

Yes, I believe you can.
And I do.

How honest are you about your needs?

There can be a self-righteous pleasure in choosing not to communicate clearly with our partners. It's a 'fuck-you' feeling that seduces us into thinking we are right and they are wrong.

At different points along the way to becoming the woman you are today, you learned the patterns of behaviour that show up time and time again in your relationship. Maybe you seek reassurance from your partner – words of affirmation that you are doing the right thing for them, or you crave for them to see how caring you are and how hard you work. Or perhaps you are frightened of being rejected if they saw the real you and in order for that not to happen, you shapeshift into versions of yourself that an Olympic gymnast would be jealous of – and then you wonder why you are so exhausted.

Whatever your background is, however you have been influenced in your life, understanding that clear communication is a gift to you and to your relationship is a fundamental piece of a healthy dynamic. Communication is king.

In the past, I would have wanted to punish my husband for not guessing what I was feeling but not speaking about. I held him to an impossible, unrealistic and, most importantly, unfair standard. Inside of me was a voice telling me that rather than it being my responsibility to speak about how I was feeling, it was somehow his responsibility to pre-empt my resentment and rage by correctly guessing what it was I was silently seething about. I would blame him for not knowing how I was feeling even though I hadn't communicated my thoughts. I thought he should have been able to pick up on the clues and respond accordingly. It was his fault for not reading the signs that I believed were obvious.

As much as I have learned about myself these last few years, I still default into old ways of being at times and, when I do, it reminds me of the importance of clear communication. We are conditioned to believe our partners should be the ones to save us, suggesting that if they knew us at all then we shouldn't have to say it, and that asking for what we want and need is selfish and ungrateful. Yet, having experienced what comes from being honest and vulnerable with my husband, I really have no time for mind games any more. If there is something that I'm thinking or feeling, I try and quieten the voice inside that makes me want to test him by waiting to see if he will get what I'm thinking based on my behaviour or attitude.

Committing to clear communication does not feed the part of me that savours the feeling of riding on my high horse. What it does instead is teach me that there is so much love and connection in being honest with my husband about how I feel. Is this worth the stomach-churning vulnerability that has to be opened up? I think it is, I really do.

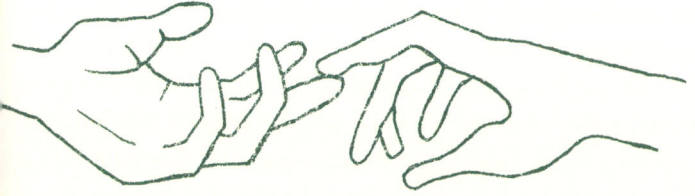

Do you have moments of pure presence?

It was 7:30 p.m. one evening. The kids were in the living room playing – I could hear them planning how best to make a cushion fort beside the couch. I stood at the kitchen sink washing the dishes we had used for dinner. The front door opened and I heard Stuart coming in, his tone of voice and happily uttered 'Hello' so normal and achingly familiar. He went into the living room and I listened as the kids vied for his attention. I could hear them scrambling to get to him and climb all over him. I drank in their laughter.

Although I continued to stand at the kitchen sink, I was no longer focused on the dishes. I was tuning in to the sounds of my life. I could feel the heartbeat of my family pulse through my whole body and, in that moment, I felt such joy in the perfection of the mundane.

I could hear Stu leaving the living room and coming into the kitchen. He came over to me and, in that moment, that sweet sweet moment, I felt the certainty of belonging. Belonging with this man, and with these kids in this life that we have built.

He stopped beside me and for a moment it was just him and me again. In that tiny second, the distance we have travelled together stretched out before me and I remembered it all.

And then the kids ran in and the moment passed. But what a moment to be alive for. Those moments are gifts. It's as though time stands still in order for us to see beyond the chaos. We get a glimpse of our why and it is magnificent.

Those moments are gifts.
It's as though time stands still
in order for us to see
beyond the chaos.

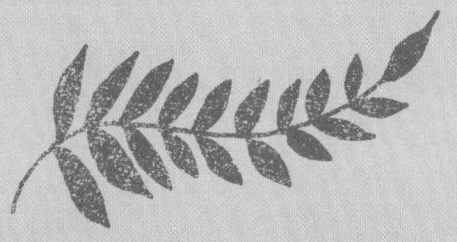

What has parenthood brought to your relationship?

I thought I knew how much he loved me then. I thought that what we had was beautiful and special and strong and built on a foundation that would see us through a lifetime. I was bursting at the seams with romantic love.

What we had then is very different to what we have now. Everything was fun and exciting back then. It was surprise weekends away, nights out and days spent lying in bed, listening to music and talking about everything and nothing, sharing hopes and ambitions for the future.

We still have fun, but it looks different now. Our conversations about our hopes and ambitions for the future started happening again when we began to emerge from the chaos that comes with those first few years of parenthood where all you're focused on is survival.

He's been at my side through my toughest times, at my back when I needed someone to help me stand and he has walked in front of me, encouraging me to take one step at a time when I couldn't see my way through the darkness.

The romantic notions of love I had are gone. They've been replaced with a much clearer understanding of what it means to love someone, to stand with them through thick and thin, to keep making your way back to each other even when the last thing you want to do is talk to the other person.

There are days that seem so mundane and yet so full of love; there are arguments that cut to the bone because tiredness has stripped away all the usual layers of defence and left us feeling exposed and vulnerable; there are differences of opinion that before would have seemed trivial but, in the current moment of 'discussion', leave us questioning if we even know each other as we thought we did. Having children has taken our relationship, chewed it up and spat it out. There is a new depth to 'us' that can only come from walking through fire together.

When you bear witness to the unravelling and rebuilding of a person, there's nothing left to the imagination and I really love that.

> I have learned that in order to love someone else, we must learn to love ourselves first.

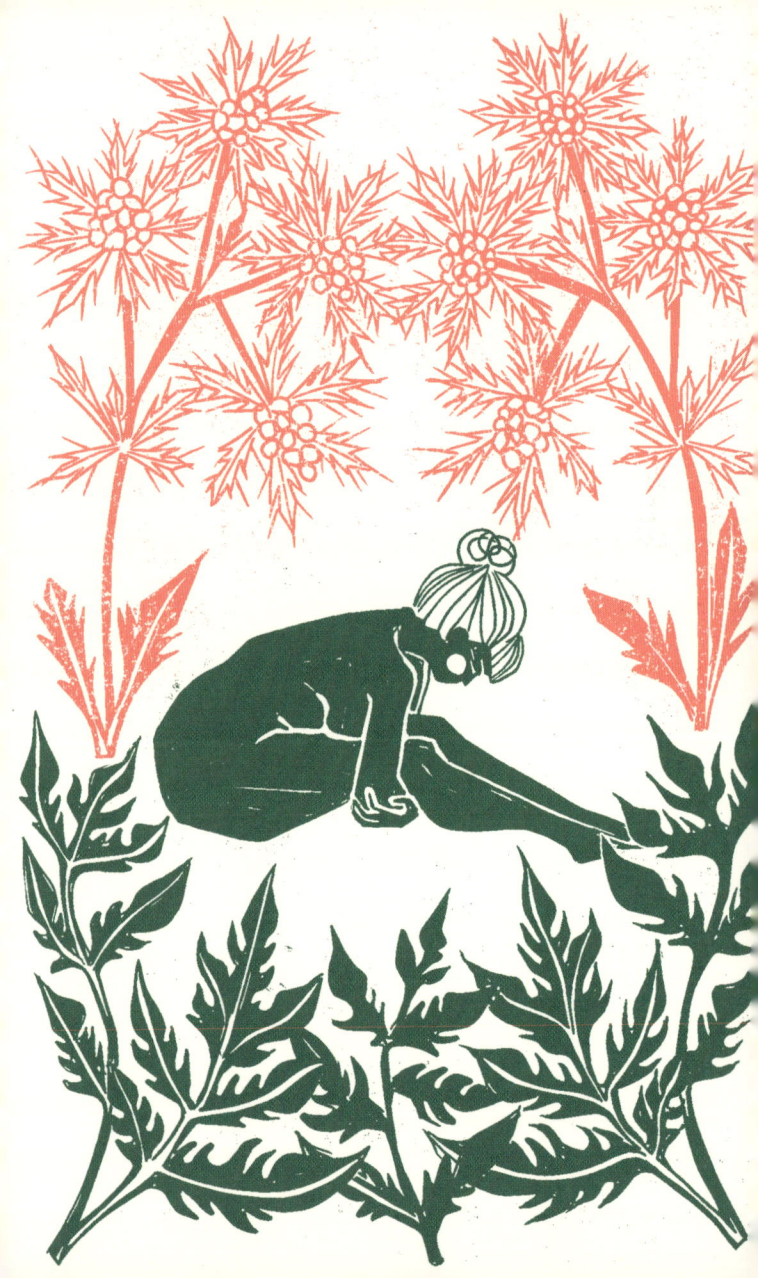

When
I lost
my
self

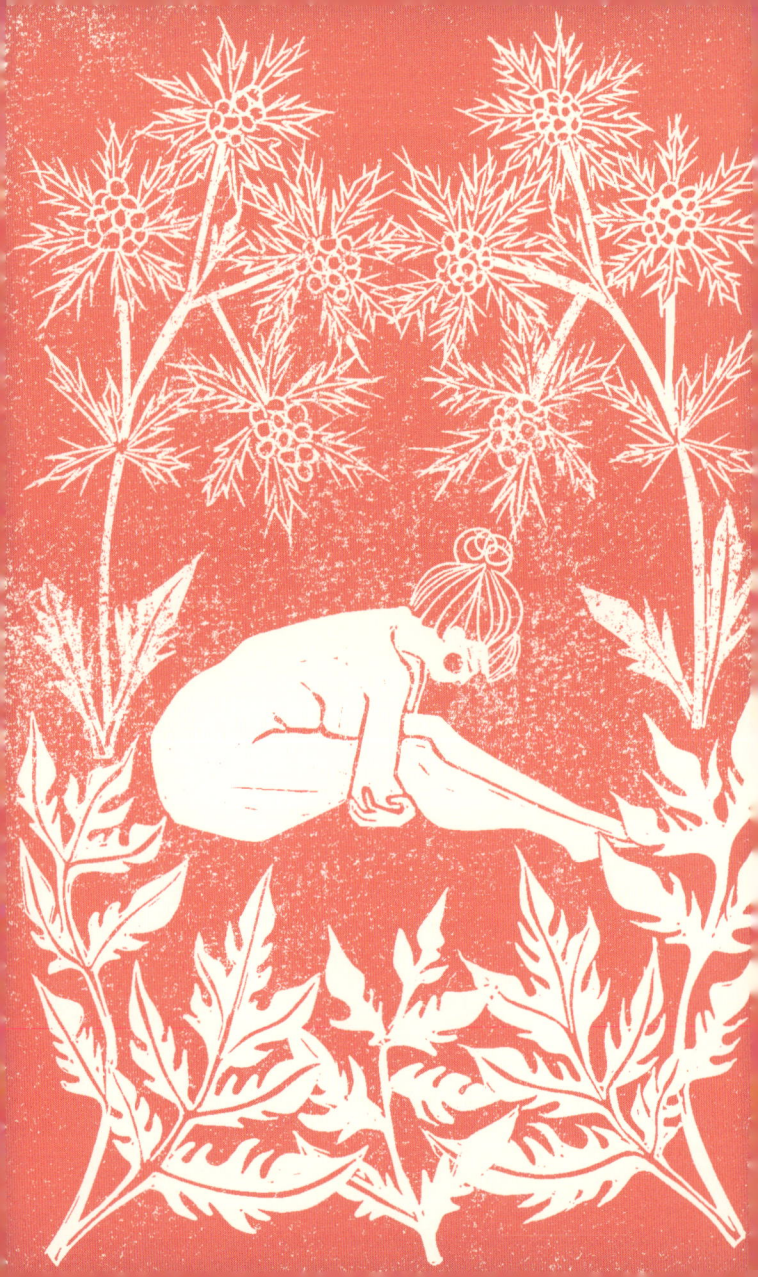

Who am I if not the woman I have always known myself to be?
Who is this version of me who stands before you today as
a mother? There is no going back to the woman we were, and we
are being lied to when they tell us that we will feel like 'ourselves'
again. No. Instead, we have to get to know who we are now, and
who we are becoming. We rob ourselves of joy when we stand
still, waiting for the ghost of who we were to sweep in and rescue
us. There is a 'dark night of the soul' in motherhood and this was
not something I had prepared for. There is a reckoning, a dying
and a rebirth of who I am. It is painful and requires facing parts of
myself that I buried long ago in shame. There are parts of my self
that motherhood will not let me run from. And that hurts. I have
to confront the parts of me that I see represented in my children.
Motherhood forces me to face myself. To find myself.
To love myself. To accept myself.

Have you tried stepping outside of 'normality'?

There's often a reluctance to leave this place you've called 'you' for so long now. Even at its most uncomfortable, it's still familiar. You tread carefully, navigating the squeaky floorboards of your emotions. You know exactly where to step to make sure you avoid the telltale creak of what's hidden there.

You tell yourself that you like it this way, that it suits you to live a half-life cleverly disguised as the perfect whole (even though you tell yourself this, you don't really believe it, do you?). I often wonder what it is that makes us so afraid to acknowledge our potential. Why do we avoid what we know will initiate change and transformation?

I think the answer to these questions is layered and nuanced and so vast that it makes my brain want to pretend to be asleep. We live in a world that teaches us that not only can the woman of today 'have it all', but she should also *want* to have it all, and that somehow it's not only our right but also our responsibility.

That is a very heavy cross to carry, my friend, especially when it's not even a cross of our own making. We are encouraged to live beyond our means. We are told we need the things they're selling, that somehow by having these things we will become better versions of ourselves. We deserve these things because 'we're worth it'.

I can't help but ask 'worth what, exactly?' Worth conforming to what other people think our lives should look and be like? We are praised for looking after ourselves, but criticized for being vain. We're brainwashed into thinking that in order to be loved we must be slim, but not too skinny. Be fun but not too loud, quirky but not weird, ambitious but not too demanding, sexy but not too sexual because 'nice' girls don't talk about their needs and wants.

We walk a very fine line and it's exhausting. We've learned what works for us. We've learned to stay within the lines. Stepping outside of this 'normality' so that you can challenge the existing structures of your life is by no means an easy feat, I know. But tolerating my own discomfort in order to appease others is not something I accept anymore.

I've stepped outside and it is beautiful.

I often **wonder** what it is that makes us so **afraid** to acknowledge our **potential.**

Who do your beliefs about motherhood serve?

The early days and weeks and months (even years) of motherhood leave us battered and bruised. So many of us emerge from that time scarred yet triumphant, bloodied and a little broken. We look around, feeling lost and alien in our environment.

It's not easy to put your finger on exactly how you feel – part of you wants to rage and scream at the difficulty that comes with the burden of motherhood. Part of you is ashamed of feeling this way. Part of you is afraid that you really are doing it all wrong because no one else seems to feel like you do. And then part of you is so madly in love that you can't even put it into words. It's so confusing to feel so torn and conflicted at the same time.

Part of you believes what you have been conditioned into thinking about motherhood. The lies and fantasies run deep, so deep we don't even know they are there until we judge other women for their motherhood. When we judge, we unearth our beliefs about other women (and ourselves). If you are looking at another mother and thinking that she can't love her children as much as you love yours because she prioritizes herself sometimes then you're touching on a belief you have about motherhood and the 'good mother'. Where does this belief come from?

You want what she seems to have. You want free time but instead of making it happen, you continue to sacrifice yourself at the altar of your family because you believe (somewhere deep down in your subconscious) that this is what a good mother does. But it doesn't stop you wanting the free time. So what do you do? You pretend that you could never do what she's doing – you love your kids too much to do that.

I'm calling it: bullshit! When you challenge the beliefs you have around motherhood, I guarantee that you won't even know where half of them come from. They're just there, running your life for you. How does that make you feel?

It made me feel uncomfortable enough to want to explore my beliefs. It made me aware of the judgements I have of other women, and it made me question these too. Where do my judgements come from? My hidden beliefs, of course. Where do these beliefs come from? Good question: childhood, school, my parents, my friends, the media, books. You name it.

Who do these beliefs serve? It's certainly not me or you.

What have you figured out about yourself and your motherhood?

It's ok to say that you're still figuring your motherhood out.

It doesn't matter if your baby was born yesterday, last week or fifty years ago. It can take a lifetime for this mantle of motherhood to settle upon us in ways that we feel comfortable with. It takes time to feel at home within ourselves when we are no longer, and never will be again, just one. Motherhood is a strange place indeed. It is full of uncertainty and newness and curiosity and adventure and heartache and unrealistic demands. There is nothing that can prepare you for the vastness that comes with motherhood – nothing.

Perhaps these early years of motherhood are the furnace in which we mothers are forged, with every challenging moment a stepping stone closer to the wiser woman of tomorrow. The mother I was when my baby was first placed in my arms is no longer the mother I am now. She exists nowhere but in the echoes of my memories and in the voice of my experience.

Like anything we become better at, it takes years of practice. The wisdom we gain does not come easy, my friend, I know. In many ways the heartache and growing pains are a rite of passage into the fulfilled and open-hearted women we dream of being one day.

This is why when you try to convince me of the terrible things you believe to be true about you right now, I don't believe you. You speak to me of your challenges. You tally up your perceived failings in front of me and then use them to justify why you feel so bad. But you can't see what I see. I see you fighting to make your way to yourself, because somewhere along the way you stopped looking within for the mother you want to be. It hurts to be so far from yourself. I see you wade through your discomfort as you relearn the confidence that is required to sift through the expectations that are piled upon you, taking only what you need and what is useful for you. I see you glow with the joy and freedom that comes when you choose to walk away from the rest of it, confident in your decisions.

I see the wisdom in your eyes that tells me more than your words ever could.

And so, together we walk, figuring our motherhoods out as we go along.

I see you **fighting** to

make your way to yourself, because

somewhere along the way

you stopped looking within for

the mother you want to be.

When will you believe you are worthy of rest?

I'll rest . . .

. . . when the toys have been picked up and organized; when I can see the floor; when the clothes have been washed, dried, folded and put away; when the beds have been changed and the toilet floor has been mopped; when the freezer is full of freshly made food; when I have my figure back to a standard that society approves of; when I'm having wild and amazing sex with my husband five times a week; when the dishes have been collected up and washed; when the kids' room is tidy . . . I'll rest when I am showered and feel fresh; when I have done my online exercise class, met up with mum friends for an energetic and sprightly walk in the park to discuss our fabulous and fun lives; when I can put my baby down for a few minutes so that I can finally get to all the things I have been too lazy to do; when I can manage my time better; when I learn how to 'balance' all the things society tells me I should be balancing; when I have my twenty-seven-second dip in the now-cold bath of self-care; when the tears blind me and I lose sight of why I feel the need to prove myself to an imaginary person.

I'll rest when I finally become a version of myself that I am currently beating myself up for not being. Only then I shall rest because only then will I feel like I deserve to rest.

I'll rest when I **finally** become a version of myself that I am currently beating myself up for not being. Only then I shall rest because only then will I feel like **I deserve to rest.**

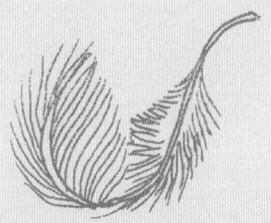

You are as **alone** as
you **think** you are.

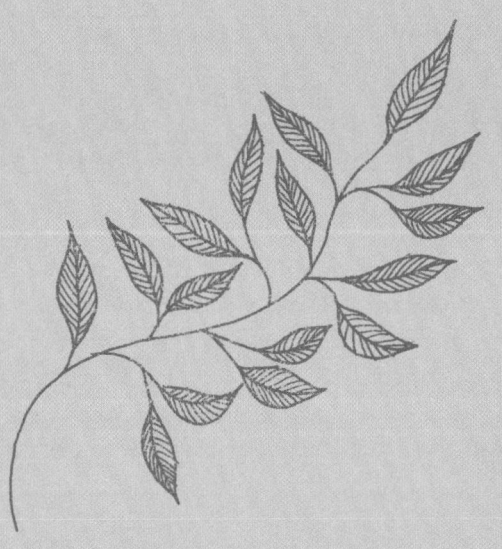

Do you think you are the only one to feel this way?

Sometimes I feel I am alone out here in the wilderness. Don't get me wrong, I'm not lost and I'm not afraid. I came here deliberately because I could not tolerate where I was.

I have found freedom here, a sense of peace and pure acceptance. Yes, I may waver in my certainty and my connection with what I know to be true, but I am only human, my friend, as are you. It took me a long time to see the beauty and the healing that exists in this place of truth. It was once a place I was frightened of, and a place that I could not imagine going to. What would I have to admit to myself in order to travel there?

You are as alone as you think you are. When you repeat to yourself that you are failing, you believe it. When you tell yourself that no other mother feels the way you do, then this is true for you.

I am here to tell you that if you embrace your truth, instead of running from it, you can find peace and acceptance.

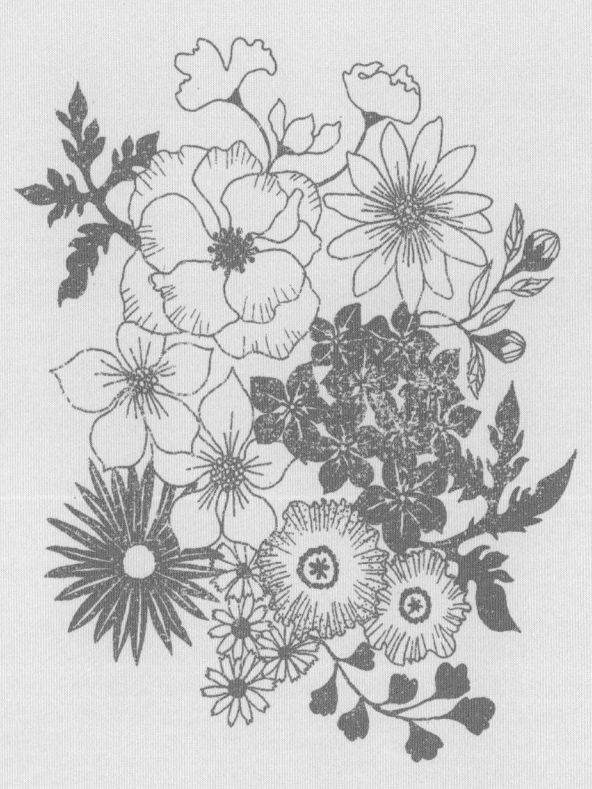

What are you not seeing?

Sometimes we can't see because we are too busy looking.
Sometimes we can't feel because we're so numb after years of ignoring our instincts.
Sometimes we can't hear because we're no longer tuned in to the frequency of our souls.
Sometimes we can't taste beauty and joy because we're choking on the words we never speak.

And then something happens. Something out of our control.
We stop looking and start seeing.
Our numbness fades and feelings rush to the surface,
new and exciting and terrifying.
We hear birds and laughter and the sweet lyrics of a song being sung by a four-year-old, and our souls weep with joy at being heard again.

Words start to spill out, words we have held in for such a long time.
Words of love and truth and hope and fear.
Words that reconnect us with ourselves and with others.
Sometimes we must trust our hearts to lead us
when all else fails.

Can you let go of all that you thought you were?

The weight of what it means to be a mother is like having the most precious and heavy stones in our pockets. Their purpose is to help us descend into the darkness for it is here that we will find ourselves.

This is a journey to the place where only mothers go.

This place exists deep, deep down inside of us and is as old as time. It is a place so sacred that in order to enter it, you must let go of all that you thought you were.

The descent can be terrifying, especially if you were not aware that such an undertaking was part of your rite of passage.

As I descended, I clung to the identity of the woman I used to be. I wrapped who I thought I was around me like a lifejacket even though she was cumbersome and ill-fitting for this stage of my life. She was the only me I had ever known. Who was I without her?

And then one day the time came where I realized that in order for me to make my way out of the darkness, I must say goodbye to the woman I was. I had to let her go with love. My soul knew that I would have to shed this skin that no longer felt like mine.

The shedding process is painful. It is a time of momentous transition where the dead parts of us, the parts that are no longer serving us, must be left behind in order that we can emerge fresh and full of vitality. This happens many times over the course of a lifetime, but none seems to have as much potency as the shedding as we transition from maiden to mother. We go from being an individual to becoming a mother, a woman who for the rest of her life will understand the unparalleled pleasure and pain that comes with bearing this title.

Detaching ourselves from who we have always known ourselves to be is not easy. Our roots run deep, and we may have mistakenly held on to her out of fear of the unknown. Who am I if I am not her? The paradox is that you will never know who you are if you don't let her go.

It's time to begin your ascent, my friend.

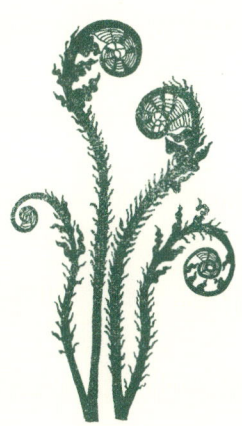

Can you reach out to others?

When I look back, I can see clearly that my early experiences of motherhood felt insecure. It was my feelings of doubt and insecurity that led me to find alternative narratives of motherhood to the ones I had been brought up on – the ones that saturated the media, and which I felt I couldn't live up to.

On a soul level, part of me knew that I had to seek others who spoke about motherhood in ways that felt true and real, for me to feel safe and secure. I sensed the inconsistencies between what I was actually experiencing and what I imagined I would experience, and it left me feeling unsure of myself.

In the beginning, my focus was all inward facing. I berated myself and told myself that it must be me who was getting it all wrong, that it must be me who was being dramatic, that it must be me who was the only woman to feel this way about motherhood.

This inward focus was hurtful, and it kept me distracted from seeing what was actually real. I believed what I was thinking, and I believed I was alone. My question was always – why is this so difficult? Also, why does everyone else seem to be managing ok and I'm not? As I began to explore these questions outside of myself, I discovered these doubts were present in the minds of so many mothers. Each of us had been staying silent, each of us believing ourselves to be the only one.

Today, years after becoming a mother, I continue to question what isn't clear to me or what makes me feel like I am failing. The difference is I now approach my discomfort and perceived inadequacies with curiosity rather than judgement for I know now that I am not alone on this adventure of self-(re)discovery.

For those of you who are in a similar situation, who perhaps feel insecure about who you are now at this stage of your life, I would encourage you to turn your self-doubt and questions outwards. Because in doing so, you will find groups of mothers just like you.

Mothers who are no longer blindly accepting of a narrative that simply isn't true for them.

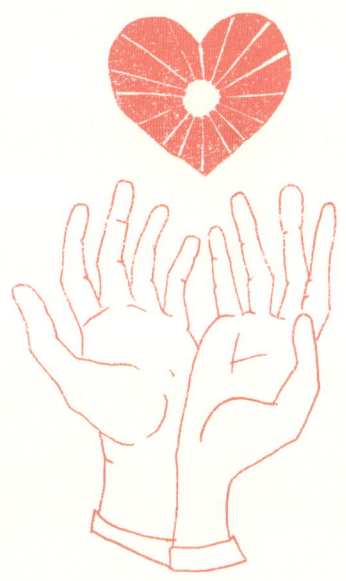

When was the last time you spoke of your pain?

'Are you there?' I asked her.

A few more seconds of silence.

'I am,' she said. 'I'm taking a moment to catch my breath because I don't want to cry over the phone with you.'

As she gathered her thoughts, I sat in silence. I closed my eyes and reminded myself that there was nothing I could say at that moment that would ease her pain, a pain I had yet to be introduced to but could feel making its way towards me.

There is pain that we deal with every day, pain that to a certain extent we have become accustomed to managing and living with. And then there is the pain that echoes through the words we use to disguise what lies beneath our veneer of being ok. This pain is both simple and complex. Simple in that we know how it feels and that it begs to be spoken about. Complex because we are making it mean something that we may be ashamed of or feel guilty about and so the thought of speaking it out loud seems like such a scary thing to do.

I know pain like this, I have some of my own. I know what it takes to open the doors to that place inside and not be sure of what will erupt, but to finally be at a point in time where you have no choice but to speak of it.

I have learned that it doesn't really help when I step into a silence that does not require me to be in the midst of it. Of course, I have done this in the past. I have immediately rushed in, believing that words of reassurance would help, that they would somehow soothe the pain that I could so clearly hear, but to be honest, felt uncomfortable with so wanted to make stop. My attempts at comforting disguised my discomfort at being faced with someone's deep and raw emotion.

The thing about being in the presence of someone's pain, is that there is really nothing we can do other than to try and stay grounded in the face of it. I have learned that when someone trusts me with their raw honesty, they are not looking for me to fix it. They may be looking for solidarity, and someone to hold on to as they try and get back on their feet but not be fixed.

How could I fix what I have not lived?

I have learned that when someone trusts me with their **raw honesty,** they are not looking for me to fix it.

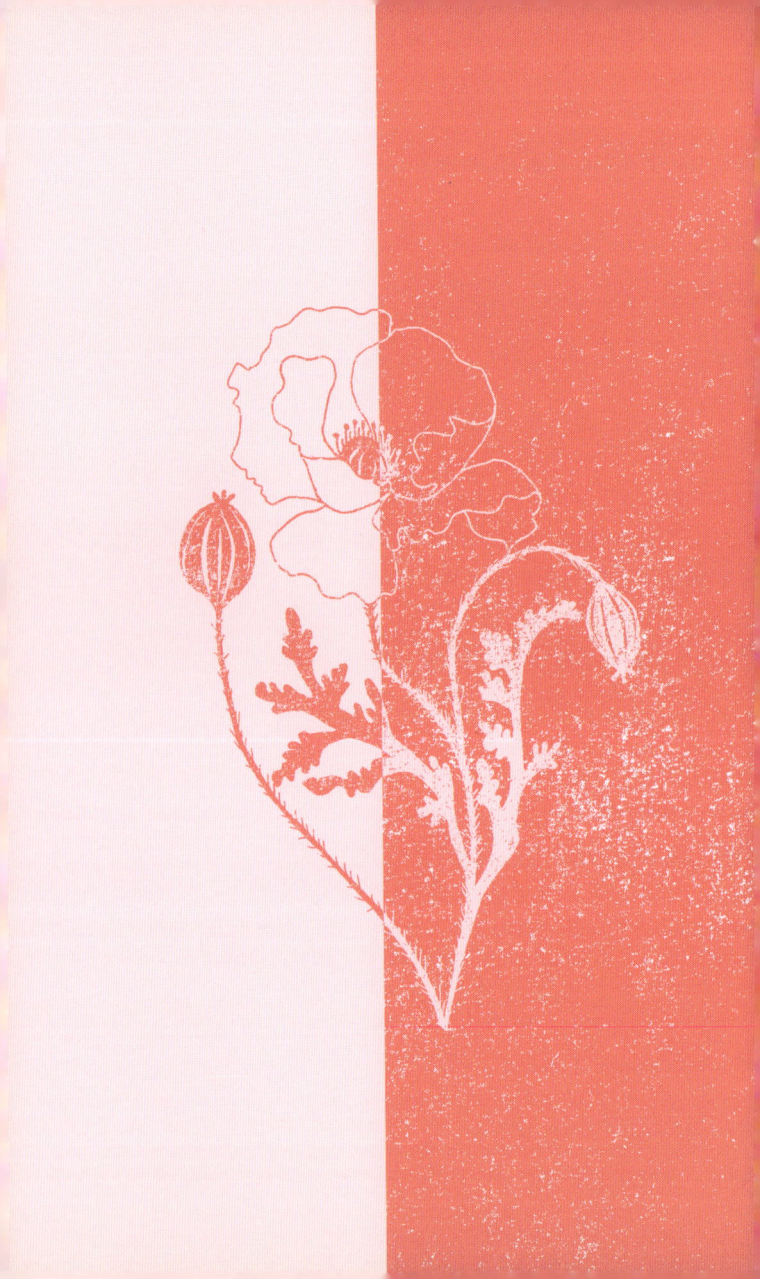

Can you feel the duality of motherhood?

One of the hardest parts of motherhood has been the recognition that I become a version of myself I find hard to bear at times. The impatience. The anger. The losing of my shit.

AND . . . one of the most healing parts of motherhood has been the recognition of how much love I have for these two little beings that are mine for a while.

The duality that exists within motherhood blows my mind.

The unparalleled pain and pleasure.

The privilege and the burden of the title 'Mammy'.

The love and the hate.

The desperation for aloneness and the hunger to see and touch my children.

Late nights and early mornings. Sorrow and joy.

Motherhood: My end and my beginning.

You will feel

the **stirrings** of

the woman you are becoming as

she **wakes** inside of you

and there will come a day when

you feel **ease** in

your life again.

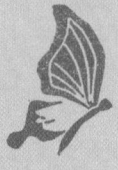
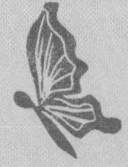

Have you ever felt frightened of losing yourself?

'I have no sense of self.'

'How am I supposed to care for myself when I have no idea who that self is?'

'Motherhood has done this. The thing I prayed for, that I have been waiting for, has taken who I thought I was and left me feeling like I don't know who I am anymore.'

All words spoken to me by a mother.

This is the part of motherhood that cannot be dressed up to look pretty. You cannot hide from this painful and soul-wrenching part of the adventure, I'm afraid. There are no Hallmark cards to celebrate the excruciating unravelling that women go through in order to become a mother who feels confident in who she is.

There is an aloneness that comes with motherhood that surprised me. It is you and you alone who has to choose to forge her way through the darkness. Other mothers wait for you. We wait because we too travelled alone at times.

I don't say this to frighten you.

I say this to send you strength, and to remind you that there are others who have walked this path in front of you and there are others finding their footing behind you. You are in a moment in time that feels like it may last forever. But it doesn't, my friend, it really doesn't.

You will feel the stirrings of the woman you are becoming as she wakes inside of you and there will come a day when you feel ease in your life again.

'But how will I survive until then?' I hear you cry.

Breath by breath, my friend. Breath by breath.

Can you find your way in the darkness?

The early years of motherhood are the perfect place for us to lose sight of ourselves. Motherhood forces us to focus on others as opposed to self. We become masters at observing and responding to cues, and we acquire exceptional skills that allow us to do things like hear a change in the breathing of our baby in the next room while we're sleeping. It is no wonder that we don't even realize we're lost. We're so busy, so dedicated to our cause, that we haven't fully realized the depth of our disconnection from self.

I only knew what it felt like to be lost because one day I went looking for the woman I was and I couldn't find her. In her place stood this magnificent mother who I somehow felt wasn't quite me. Her voice, the way she spoke, her priorities and her confidence in dealing with her babies astounded me. Is this me? Am I her? How can this be? When did I end and she begin?

In the early years of my motherhood, there were times when I felt like I was stumbling in a maze of dark passageways. Yes, I had purpose. Yes, I was in love. But I also felt alone and lost. I felt like an echo of the woman I had been.

I know the uneven floors of the dark passageways you feel trapped in. I know every inch of them. I have run my fingers along every crack and crevice in the walls, lacerating my skin and heart in the process, desperately seeking something but uncertain of what exactly it was.

And then one day I found what I had been looking for.
I found the footprints left behind by the women who had walked these dark passages before me. At first I didn't believe that I wasn't alone, that it wasn't just me. I decided to look for the next footprint, and the next one after that. And before I knew it, I had found a way forward and my journey to myself had begun. I made sure to stamp my footprints into the ground, because I wanted to be sure that they would be found by the women who were coming after me.

And so, my friend, if you have stumbled upon my footprint, I hope you know that even in the darkest of moments, even when you feel like there is no end to these dark passageways, you are not alone.

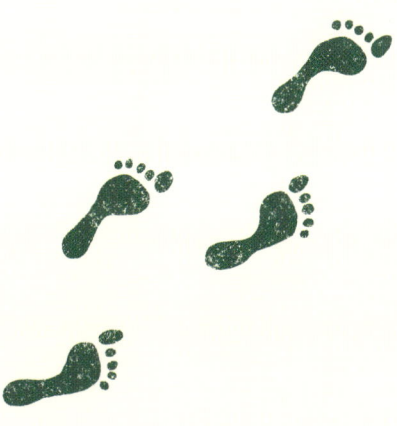

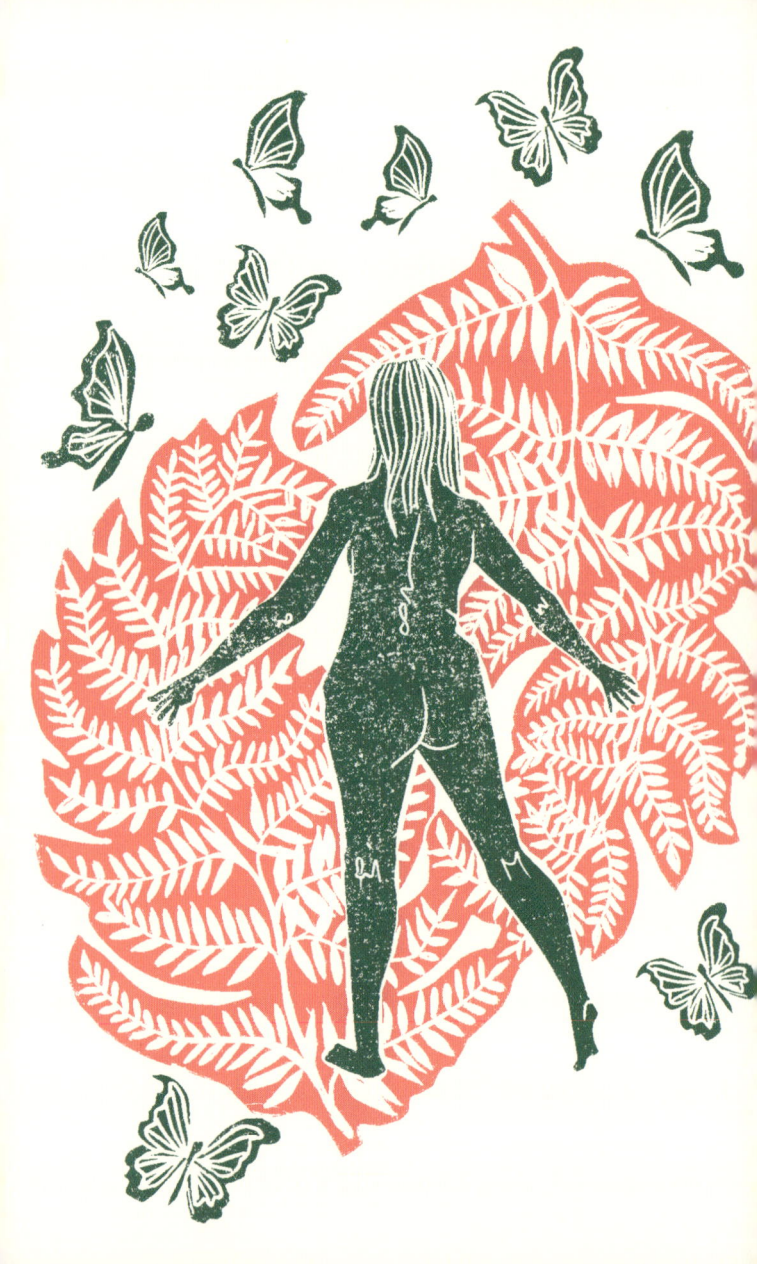

My self, my strength

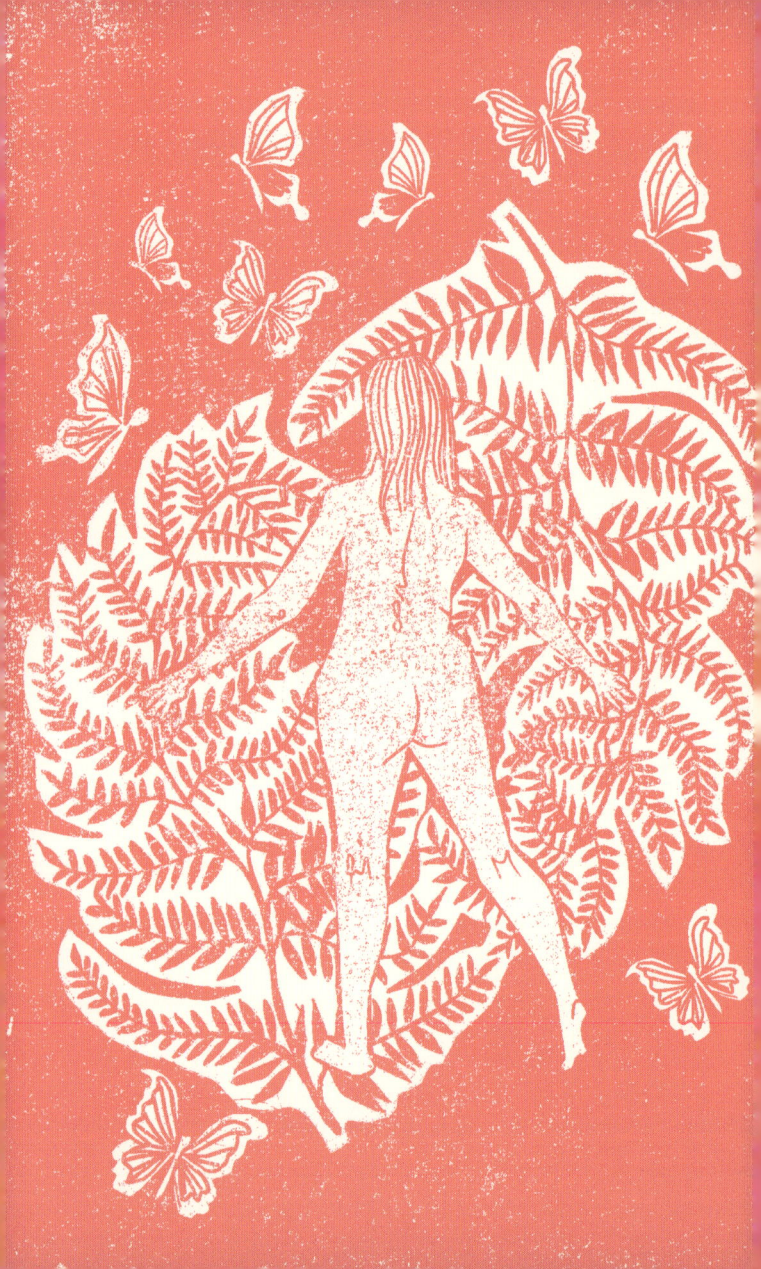

Motherhood brings out the very best and the very worst of me. I have learned this about myself on my adventures into the wilderness of my life. I am at my most beautiful and my ugliest when I am in the throes of the joy and rage that only a mother feels.

I have never loved as much or as deeply since I became a mother. At times I am terrified by the magnitude of what it means to love so much because I know this love means the annihilation of my heart and soul if my worst nightmares were to come true.

So I have to choose to bring myself back to the place of incredible love. To anchor myself in the here and now and trust that if this is all I get then I am one of the luckiest women alive.

There are moments of pure awe in my life and they catch me by surprise when they come. They can never be called upon – they don't work like that. It's almost as if they drop in like a gift from somewhere magical, somewhere that can't be defined but is full of love. A reminder of how incredible a mother I am in the midst of all my self-doubt.

These moments whisper for me to look, to be silent, and take it all in. To feel them and breathe them. They ask me to open my heart and allow this truth to pierce the lies I have told myself about who I am as a mother.

I allow these truths to wash over me.

I drink my fill of the beautiful moment and in that sacred stillness, I believe that I am an incredible mother to my children.

I believe it.

May you too be open to those moments of awe, my friend.

Do you know this feeling I speak of?

When you look at your life, what do you see? What do you feel? What sounds do you hear? What does it taste like?

Sometimes, we can't see the beauty and perfection in what we have because we think such things only come as a result of a concentrated and orchestrated effort at making them happen. This is what we're taught to believe: that everything we want, everything we dream of, is just slightly out of reach. Be better and you'll get better. Do more and you'll have more. We don't know the progress we're making when we've got our heads down in the midst of it. We can't see the bigger picture when we're so focused on honing our skills and changing old habits.

Yes, we can lift our heads, search the horizon and make sure we're still heading in the direction of our dreams but we don't often notice how far we've actually come. It's not until we are far enough away from where we started that we can look back and see how far we've come.

Has the journey been hard? Yes.

Did we want to quit sometimes? Also yes.

Is it worth it? Hell, yes!

Keep putting one foot in front of the other. Look at what you can control. Remind yourself why you're doing this. Remember to breathe. No one can do this for you, but, side by side, we've got this.

This is true for all of us. When we're busy transforming, we can't see the shedding that takes place, we can't see the momentum that we create every time we choose to live in alignment with who we actually are and not who we think we should be.

But we can feel it.

It feels like ease and acceptance. It feels like certainty in the face of doubt. It feels like settling back into a version of yourself that has been waiting for you to come home.

This is what

we're taught to believe:

that everything we want,

everything we dream of,

is just slightly out

of reach.

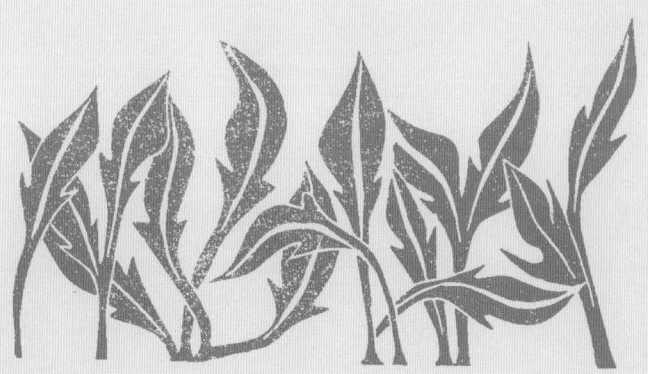

What fears do you have?

I talk a lot about fears with the mums I work with. We hold hands and we go exploring among their thoughts. We dust off old values and belief-structures to see why they think the way they do (spoiler alert: we often think the way we do because that's what our parents thought, or our teachers told us, and so on . . .).

We start poking around in the feelings they have, the reasons why things are the way they are for them. We start dismantling opinions and 'just because' statements. After digging for a while, we get to a point where we hit something solid: deeply hidden but powerful beliefs like 'I'm not good enough'. But rather than keep going, there is an attempt to circle back and go in the other direction because the gold we've just hit is too painful, awkward and uncomfortable to acknowledge.

You look at other people and see their lives brimming with potential, possibility and promise. You want that in your life but think it's never going to happen. And so you end up accepting where you are or surrendering to what you know to be true for you, pretending that everything is fine but continuing to lie awake at night, feeling that gnawing hunger in your soul that cannot be lied to. You choose to prioritize 'fitting in' but are not able to look at yourself in the mirror because you can't accept what you see. You resist the 'what if' and resign yourself to the 'this is just the way it is'.

Where did you learn that all of you, your greatness and your potential, were things to be afraid of? When did you learn to settle for a half-lived life? What do you fear will happen if you tune in to the part of you that tells you there is more? Imagine if you unearthed your fears and examined them with a heart full of wonder and curiosity instead of looking away in fear?

Treasure is rarely stumbled upon. It's more often searched for, dived for or dug deep for. What makes the treasure inside of you any different? And it is treasure, all of it. Every last doubt and fear is there for you to learn from, to appreciate and eventually love for what it can teach you if you would just let it.

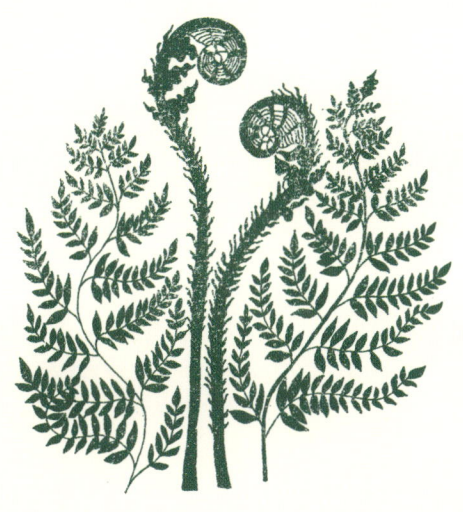

Do you lie to yourself?

How finely tuned is your bullshit detector? What would you give it out of ten? Mine has always been pretty good (let's call it an eight out of ten), but so too has been my ability to ignore it and try to pretend that the deep thoughts and unsettled feelings I have that whisper and pull at me are nothing to be concerned about. (Pretending to myself? Come on! How exhausting and ridiculous is that?)

Who are you trying to kid? No, really. Have you ever actually thought about who you are trying to kid? I ask myself this same question – it's a tough but good one. You know it's pointless to try and kid yourself, so who is it? And why? What image of yourself are you trying to maintain and in whose eyes?

Now that we're here, together in this space, let's keep going with this. What is it you're afraid of? What is it about your truth that you're reluctant to face? Because the reality is we all know that when our words and actions don't align with our thoughts, we feel the tension, and we suffer the discomfort that arises from not being congruent with who we know we are meant to be.

Whenever I detect my bullshit detector hits that sweet spot of ten out of ten (ding, ding, ding), it's usually because I'm trying to dodge responsibility in some shape or form. Maybe it's something small like staying accountable and making a phone call that I said I would make or maybe it looks like me not facing up to what needs to be done because I think it's going to be uncomfortable or awkward or difficult or whatever . . . it doesn't really matter, does it? The results are the same.

The more we quieten and dim and smother those thoughts and feelings, the more pungent their decay becomes. Ahhh . . . that sweet, familiar stench.

So tell me, if your BS detector could talk, what score out of ten would it give itself?

What **image** of yourself are you trying to **maintain** and in whose **eyes**?

What's your relationship with loneliness?

It's a strange place to be when you feel untethered to your own life. You look around and marvel at the wonders you have achieved, the relationships you have cultivated and yet still feel an ache, and a sense of loneliness that no one and no thing can soothe.

To feel lonely hurts. To be surrounded by people who like you, or even a person who loves you, and still feel lonely speaks to something bigger than the company of others being the solution. The extent to which loneliness is a part of motherhood has been kept hidden. It is something not spoken about because it doesn't fit with the ideology of motherhood being all-fulfilling for those who embark on its adventure.

There is a loneliness in motherhood that is soul deep. No amount of company or coffee mornings can keep it at bay and this makes me wonder if our loneliness is something we must learn to overcome, a challenge to be gently and strongly faced as we venture deeper into the woman and mother we are becoming. It requires getting comfortable with being uncomfortable.
It means being able to sit with your loneliness, and to not run from the pain it brings because part of you knows that in order for you to keep moving forward in your motherhood, you must face this part of you – the part that is letting go and detaching from an old life, old friends and an old way of being. To let go means that for a while you are untethered. You are neither here nor there and that can be a terrifying place to be.

I no longer fit where I used to belong and I have not yet carved my place in my new environment for I still wander. There are personal battles to be won and wars that are waged in the pursuit of understanding why loneliness is so ever present in motherhood. I think part of this achievement can only be arrived at as a result of going inwards during our loneliness.

And often it is not until the loneliness you felt has gone, the loneliness that frightened and hurt you, that you realize that you have made it through. You have overcome this obstacle and now find yourself in a new stage of your motherhood – a stage where you are feeling more confident in yourself and your abilities as a mother. These are hard-won accomplishments and no one can do them for you.

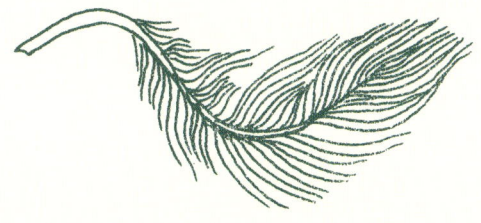

Have you considered letting your light shine?

When we are in darkness and feel what we cannot see, this is also when we have the potential to shine our brightest. This is when the tiniest of embers and the smallest of glimmers can make the biggest difference. The most wonderful thing about darkness is when it gets lit up.

There have been times in my life when I felt like I was engulfed by darkness. I felt like my light had been wiped out or turned off. There have been times when I chose to dim my own light because I did not want to face the reality of my life and so I retreated to darkness to lick my wounds.

I went seeking the light from others because I felt that if I could just get some of what other people had I would feel better, and I would be able to get by without reigniting myself again. I chased the dawn because it gave me hope but I was not prepared to meet it head on with the light that can only come from within. I wanted to take but not commit. I wanted sustenance but not nourishment. I was getting by but not really living.

Yes, we can warm our hands from the light of a fire, and we can take shelter from those around us who have enough light for two or three people at a time. We can even sit under the stars and be in awe of how brightly they shine. But this is not enough.

A soul cannot dance without expressing its light. We can starve ourselves of our light, and we can make every attempt to stifle the magnificence of our uniqueness but we cannot live like this without consequence. When you compare yourself to others, you dampen your light. When you think that who you are is not good enough, you stifle more of your light. When you believe poisonous rhetoric about what makes a person beautiful, your light dims a little more.

You are not here to compare yourself. It is not possible to compare the incomparable. There is no one like you. There never has been and there never will be again. The light that is inside of you is once in a lifetime. Do not be afraid to let it shine.

Sometimes you forget that just as you have sought sustenance and shelter from the light of others, others too are looking to be reassured by your light.

We need you to be the light of your own life.

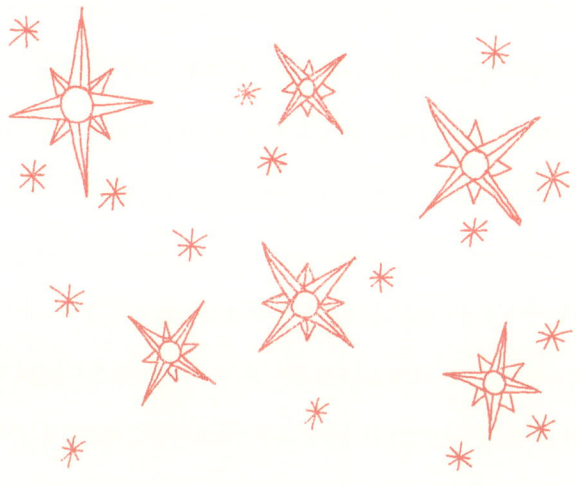

Can you let go of the idea of perfection?

As mothers we are encouraged to embody perfection and comparison as if it's a 'normal' thing to do. But I no longer choose to be part of this damaging paradigm of motherhood. Since becoming a mother, I have found myself in spaces and conversations I never knew existed. I have walked through fire searching for connection with mothers who felt the same. I have whispered and written, spoken and roared about how we are being failed as mothers in the hope that another mother, somewhere, would hear my battle cry.

The truth of 'motherhood' is so far from the pettiness of 'comparison' that it hurts to use both words in the same sentence. Motherhood is a fierce and unforgiving force. It reaches into the depth of our souls and it claws and tears at the sacred parts of us that are buried deep, deep down inside. It fights to expose our pulsating vulnerabilities. It needs to tap into and feed off them in order to teach and remind us that we are powerful beyond anything we can imagine. It yanks and pulls these precious parts of us through our bodies, and it gives birth to a strength that we could never have imagined possessing. It is the strength of a warrior. It is a strength that legends are made of. It is the strength of a mother.

If motherhood could whisper in our ear, I imagine it would tell us to stop being scared of stepping into its void; to trust that it will catch us, if we would only leap. It would tell us fables of brave, beautiful, unicorn women who knew comparison and perfection for what they were – thieves created to trap us and keep us distracted by the external rather than discovering who we really are and what matters to us.

Your motherhood is yours. In order to surrender to it, you must give yourself permission to embrace all of its beauty and rawness. Perhaps you might give yourself permission to love yourself, even on the days when you fall for the lie that you don't deserve to be loved as you are. Rise to the challenges knowing that you are only able to do so because your feet can push off rock-bottom.

Perfection exists nowhere except in the standards that are a lie. The truth is you, as you are.

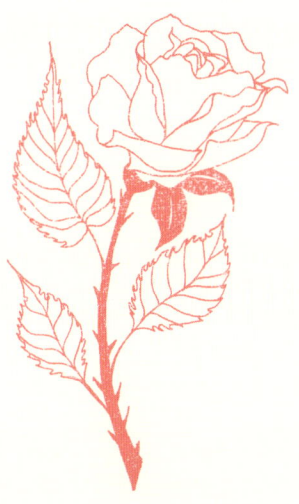

Anything can happen
and this is as terrifying as
it is reassuring.

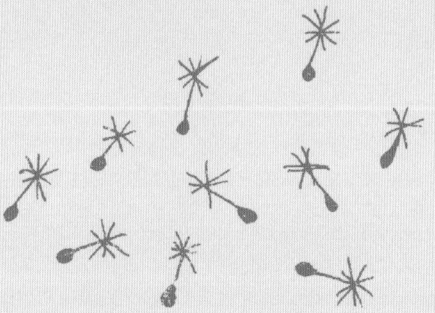

What do you need right now for the moment you are in?

Everyone has pain. Everyone is carrying their own versions of hell around with them.
We all have prisons of shame and guilt.
We all think our own is the worst.
We've all begged for something to be different in a moment of time. Please God, don't let this be true, don't let this be happening.
We've all experienced moments of joy. Feelings of happiness so pure have run through our veins that we thought we would burst from the joy it brought.
We all question who we are, what we are doing and whether or not we are making a difference in this world or doing a good job.
We've all fallen asleep to the whispering of our mind asking us if we did enough that day to make our children feel loved.
Everyone has stood strong at some point in their lives when others needed a place to take shelter from the storms that were ravaging their lives.
Everyone has lain on the ground wondering if they will ever get back up again.
There is no escaping grief and loss. You cannot hide from fear.
The thing you love the most is what will cause you the most pain.
Love makes your heart sing in joy and in sorrow.
I am still learning what it means to be alive because there are no rules to this thing we call life. Anything can happen and this is as terrifying as it is reassuring.
Sending love for the moment in time you are in when you read this.

How prepared are you to challenge your own stories?

It is hard work to raise our children so that they see us as more than the woman they call mother who does everything for everyone. It is hard work to teach our children that there is nothing wrong or selfish in claiming time for ourselves. In fact, perhaps in showing them that we are human, and that we have needs and breaking points, we are giving them a gift that no perfect mother can. The gift of humanity.

The way I live my life teaches my daughter that she need not be a slave to the demands of her family. The way I live my life teaches my son that the women in his life are to be supported in their dreams as much as he is supported in his.

Your ability to be real is what makes you spectacular at what you do. Your reserves of love can only carry you so far, and after that you become emptier and emptier of all that you are. Our children do not ask this of us. My children have never asked me to sacrifice my dreams or myself for them. No, it is the poisonous tentacles of outdated societal structures that ask this of us.

Those who truly love you and want the best for you will not require you to continually put yourself last and at the bottom of the list for everything. They may have become used to this way of life but they don't actually ask it of you. This is where your commitment to self comes in.

Are you prepared to challenge your own stories?

Are you prepared to begin the process of change in your family so that your children can watch and learn from a woman who is figuring out how to love herself enough to make space for her dreams?

Because this is how all transformations start. Not with me but with you acknowledging to yourself first that you're no longer prepared to stay where you are.

Stay the same or expand. You get to choose.

Your ability to

be **real**

is what makes you

spectacular

at what you do.

Have you appointed yourself as the sacrificial lamb in your family?

'What's more important than me, Mammy?' my daughter asked.

I looked at her and she was looking at me and her question wasn't harsh or accusatory. It was curious. She was curious. We were in the kitchen. I was at the table working and she asked me to help her find something. I told her I was finishing up some important work and then I would play with her. This is when she asked her question. I bit my tongue to stop the words that wanted to rush out of my mouth. I wanted to proclaim that nothing was more important – but that's not true. It would have been a knee-jerk platitude.

She is without a doubt one of the most important things in my life, as is my son. But I don't want to contribute to the paradigm of motherhood that promotes selflessness as the pinnacle of motherhood. I've spent too long trying to challenge it! I don't want to guilt myself into responding immediately when there is no need for it.

Nowadays, I refuse to be the self-appointed sacrificial lamb in my family – no one demands or expects it except me. I am my own persecutor, and my own jailer. I'm the one who has lit fires under myself, all the while complaining about the heat.

It has taken time for me to unravel the beliefs I have around motherhood and the role a mother plays in the family. There have been a lot of ups and downs as my husband and I found the words to talk about what we felt was happening in our family unit, and how frustrated, shocked and stressed we sometimes were at how we had slid into such stereotypical gender roles since our children arrived. He is my biggest supporter and advocate (as I am his) and we have had some challenging conversations about how we found ourselves knee-deep in roles we never imagined would happen to us.

And so, to answer your question, my darling girl. There are people in my life who are as important as you – me being one of them. I hope one day, if you are faced with the reality of lighting a fire under yourself in the name of motherhood, you will remember that your mammy taught you to set fire to the opinions of others instead.

Have you found motherhood to be a lonely place?

Motherhood can be a frighteningly lonely experience.

It seems to initiate a time of reckoning for a lot of mums and I include myself in this. There are some mums who evolve beautifully and seemingly with ease into this phase of their lives, and then there are others who feel like they cannot breathe with the intensity of the demands placed upon them. Many remain silent about the growing burden of disconnect and withdraw from those around them for fear of being seen as not coping.

We allow our perceptions of what others are thinking about us, and the decisions we make, to fester and grow in our minds, to the point that they burrow down so deeply we can no longer see what's real and what's not. Society plays a huge role in the continued downplaying of the role of a mother. We are shamed for 'inappropriate' behaviour that is deemed unsuitable for a mother, we are shamed for how we give birth and we are made to feel lacking if we don't live up to some shadowy, idealistic, all-singing-all-dancing paragon of motherhood. Why has it become acceptable to speak the words 'I'm JUST a mum?' There is no 'just' about being a mum.

There is you. The woman who has stayed awake all night for fear of not hearing the baby if she cries. The woman who with the touch of her hand and the sound of her voice, brings so much comfort, love and security. The woman who is home. Not the house, not the town, not the country. It's you. You are the one who is home to your little ones.

There is you. The woman who has cried in the shower because even though she felt like she couldn't make it through another day, she did because she knew there was no other choice.

There is you. The woman who has fought for what she knows her child is entitled to: a fair start in life and a chance to be all they can be.

There is only you.

There will only ever be you.

I have seen you at your best and I have held you at your worst because you are me. We are one and the same, you and I.

There is nothing 'just' about us.

> I have seen you at your **best** and I have held you at your **worst** because you are me.

Do you give so much of yourself that you feel empty at times?

You are not here to give so much of yourself that you are left feeling empty.
You are not here to run yourself into the ground rather than face the discomfort of communicating your needs.
You are not here to make yourself sick because you are denying yourself the time alone that you are desperately craving.
You are not here to sacrifice everything for your family.
You are not here to live with the knowledge that you consistently value others over yourself.
You are not here to know all the answers in your motherhood.
You are not here to teach your children that becoming a mother equates to a life of servitude and self-sacrifice.

Perhaps part of why we are here is to try and embody the paradoxical privilege of what it means to be a mother, and to surrender to the ferocious love that swamps us when we think of our children, and to learn how to be part of it rather than fight it.

There are times when the woman in me battles for priority over the mother in me; they each rage a private war inside of me, and my heart and soul are the landscapes on which they battle. I've not yet fully learned the intricacies of merging both these parts of my self – perhaps they'll spend a lifetime weaving in and out of each other, forever entwined and yet separate.

Maybe that's the way of it.

But I am here for the teaching. I am here for that.

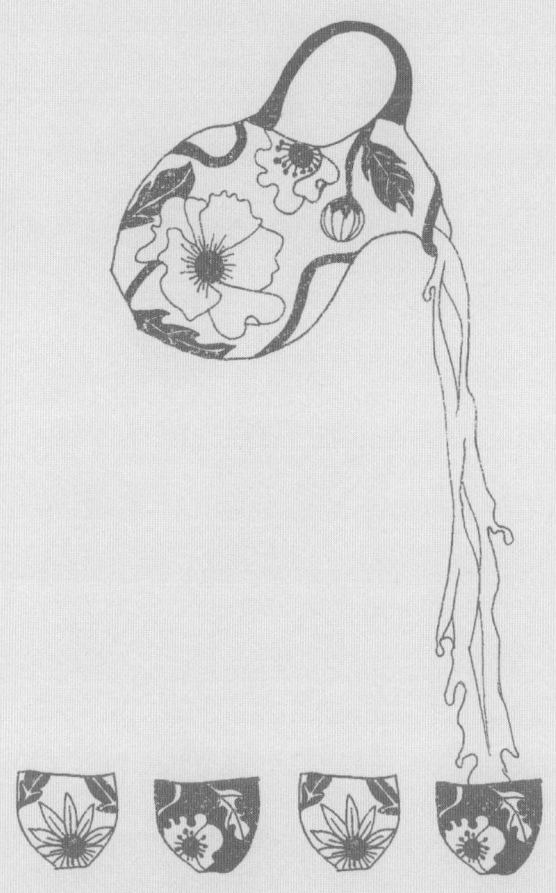

Have you noticed how motherhood has changed you?

Do not be afraid of what you know to be true for you even when it feels like you are different.
Do not let the outdated narratives of motherhood that caged our mothers and our grandmothers continue to cage you.
Do not buy into the fantasy that we are supposed to enjoy every moment of motherhood.
Do not be afraid to challenge your own deeply held beliefs as to what makes a good mother.
Do not be afraid to redefine your motherhood because in doing so, you have an opportunity to create something that is as beautiful and as unique as you.
Motherhood changes us.
Do not be afraid of that.

Mental Health Resources

UK

Maternal Mental Health Alliance (MMHA) - Empowering parents and those around them, with mental health knowledge before, during and after pregnancy.
https://maternalmentalhealthalliance.org/about-us

MumsAid –Award-winning charity providing pregnant women and new mums with specialist counselling for emotional or mental health difficulties. Their vision is of a society where all mothers are supported to give their babies the best start in life.
https://www.mums-aid.org

Mind - Perinatal mental health support and services. If you're experiencing a mental health problem in pregnancy or after having a baby, you aren't alone. Services and organizations exist to support you.
https://www.mind.org.uk

PANDAS – Community offering peer-to-peer support for you, your family and your network. PANDAS is there, whatever the weather, to offer hope, empathy and support for every parent or network affected by perinatal mental illness.
https://pandasfoundation.org.uk

Ireland

Nurture Health - Professional counselling support services to women and partners, navigating all aspects of pregnancy, fertility, childbirth, loss, perimenopause and menopause.
https://nurturehealth.ie

HSE Specialist Perinatal Mental Health Services – Hub/spoke model in all maternity units. Includes online video care and downloadable info leaflets.
www.hse.ie/eng/services/list/4/mental-health-services/specialist-perinatal-mental-health

Parentline – National, confidential helpline that offers parents support, information and guidance on all aspects of being a parent and any parenting issues.
https://parentline.ie | tel: 018733500

USA

Postpartum Support International - Promoting awareness, prevention and treatment of mental health issues related to childbearing in every country worldwide.
https://postpartum.net/get-help

The Postpartum Stress Center - Treatment and professional training center for prenatal and postpartum depression and anxiety. It also offers a full range of general counseling services to individuals or couples seeking support.
www.postpartumstress.com

Further Reading

A Life's Work by Rachel Cusk

Fair Play by Eve Rodsky

Intensive Mothering: The Cultural Contradictions of Modern Motherhood by Linda Rose Ennis

Matricentric Feminism: Theory, Activism, Practice by Dr. Andrea O'Reilly

Mom Rage: The Everyday Crisis of Modern Motherhood by Minna Dubin

Motherhood: Facing and Finding Yourself by Lisa Marchiano

Of Woman Born: Motherhood as Experience and Institution by Adrienne Rich

Revolutionary Mothering: Love On The Front Lines, edited by Alexis Pauline Gumbs, China Martens and Mai'a Williams

Silencing The Self: Woman and Depression by Dana Crowley Jack

The Mask of Motherhood: How Becoming a Mother Changes Everything and Why We Pretend it Doesn't by Susan Maushart

Torn In Two: Maternal Ambivalence by Rozsika Parker

About the author

Jacqueline Kelly is a psychotherapist and matrescence coach who has been supporting mums since 2018 and running courses for women struggling with the loss of self in motherhood. She lives in Dublin with her husband and two children. This is her first book.

About the illustrator

Rosie Lovelock is an artist and printmaker working in South East London. Her main practice is lino print – using line and pattern to carve out beautiful designs with a focus on botanical shapes and the female form.

Her interest in stories has shaped the way she approaches her work, finding a meaningful narrative in the images she makes.

Quarto

First published in 2026
by Leaping Hare Press
an imprint of The Quarto Group.
One Triptych Place, London,
SE1 9SH,
United Kingdom
T (0)20 7700 9000
www.Quarto.com

EEA Representation, WTS Tax d.o.o., Žanova ulica 3, 4000 Kranj, Slovenia
www.wts-tax.si

Text Copyright © 2026 Jacqueline Kelly
Illustration Copyright © 2026 Rosie Lovelock
Design Copyright © 2026 Quarto Publishing plc

Jacqueline Kelly has asserted her moral right to be identified as the Author of this Work in accordance with the Copyright Designs and Patents Act 1988.

All rights reserved. No part of this book may be reproduced or utilised in any form or by any means, electronic or mechanical, including photocopying, recording or by any information storage and retrieval system, without permission in writing from Leaping Hare Press.

Every effort has been made to trace the copyright holders of material quoted in this book. If application is made in writing to the publisher, any omissions will be included in future editions.

A catalogue record for this book is available from the British Library.

ISBN 978-1-83600-759-3
Ebook ISBN 978-1-83600-760-9

10 9 8 7 6 5 4 3 2 1

Design by Hanri van Wyk

Commissioning Editor: Sophie Lazar
Senior Editor: Nicky Hill
Senior Designer: Renata Latipova
Senior Production Controller: Rohana Yusof
Illustrator: Rosie Lovelock

Printed in Guangdong, China TT/Nov/2025

MIX
Paper | Supporting
responsible forestry
FSC® C016973

> The information in this book should not be treated as a substitute for professional counselling or medical advice. Any use of the information in this book is at the reader's discretion and risk.